Big Pharma Says You Have ADHD!

Dr. Jerry D. Smith Jr., PsyD, LP, LSOTP, ADHD-PT

Breakthrough Psychological Solutions PLLC

Dedication

To Kara,

For your unwavering support, boundless patience, and the love that lights every page of this journey. This book, much like every chapter of my life, is profoundly enriched and beautifully illuminated by your presence. Thank you for being my steadfast companion and my confidant. This endeavor, and all that I am, flourish under the sunshine of your love.

With all my heart,

Jerry

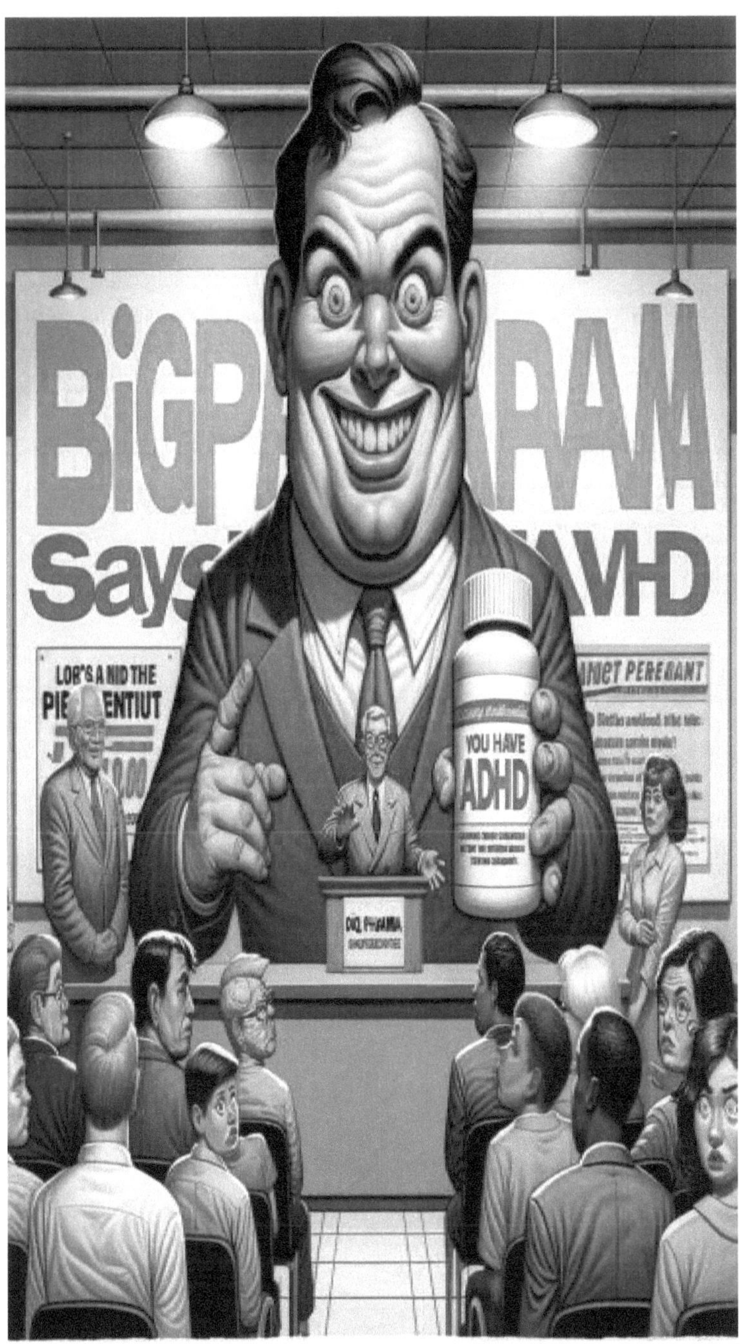

BiGPHARMA
Says
ADHD
YOU HAVE
ADHD

Introduction

In a world increasingly driven by the influence of powerful corporations, understanding the intricate dynamics between these entities and our everyday lives is more crucial than ever. This book, through a blend of anecdotes, dazzling illustrations, and thorough research, delves into one of the most pervasive and controversial mental health topics of our time: the role of Big Pharma in shaping the narrative around Attention Deficit Hyperactivity Disorder (ADHD).

The Tale of Daydreaming Danny and the Mysterious Marketing Magicians opens the gateway to this exploration. Here, we meet Danny, whose story sets the stage for Chapter 1, "How Big Pharma Shapes the ADHD Narrative." This chapter uncovers the complex web of influence woven by pharmaceutical companies in defining and disseminating information about ADHD, a condition that has increasingly found its way into the public consciousness.

In **The Curious Case of Greg and the "Distract-a-lot" Syndrome**, we encounter a narrative that leads into Chapter 2, "Big Pharma's Influence on ADHD Awareness Campaigns." This segment reveals how pharmaceutical companies don't just market drugs, but also conditions, significantly impacting public and professional understanding of ADHD.

Chapter 3, "Pharma and the Medicalization of ADHD," is prefaced by **Dr. Green's "Mysterious" Change of Heart**. This anecdote illustrates how medical professionals' perspectives on ADHD can be influenced, consciously or unconsciously, by the pharmaceutical industry's outreach and educational efforts.

Dr. Larry and the Great "Sneezitis" Epidemic humorously introduces Chapter 4, "Shaping the Definition - Big Pharma's Influence on Diagnostic Criteria." This part of the book investigates how pharmaceutical companies play a role in defining what ADHD is and isn't, influencing both diagnosis and treatment.

In **Tim's Enlightening Journey to the "Chronic Distraction Disorder" Diagnosis**, we embark on a path that leads to Chapter 5, "Selling Sickness - The Risks of DTC (Direct-to-Consumer) Advertising." This chapter evaluates the impact of DTC advertising on public perception and the potential risks of this form of marketing, especially in the context of ADHD.

Chapter 6, "Advocating for Big Pharma - The Influence of Industry Partnerships," is set up by **The Great Guacamole Gala of 2023**. This story uncovers the often-unseen world of industry partnerships and their influence on public health agendas and research priorities.

In **Dr. Monty and the Mysteriously Appearing Muffin Baskets**, we find an entry point into Chapter 7, "Crafting the Message - Pharma's Influence on Healthcare Providers." This chapter examines the methods used by pharmaceutical companies to sway the opinions and prescribing habits of healthcare providers.

The Curious Case of Bubbly Billy in Bhutan introduces Chapter 8, "Expanding Markets - Big Pharma's Global Influence." This chapter expands the discussion beyond domestic borders, exploring how pharmaceutical companies shape ADHD narratives and treatment practices globally.

Dr. Phil McCrackin's Wild Ride with "PillPal" Promos sets the stage for Chapter 9, "Limiting Big Pharma's Influence through Regulation." This chapter discusses the regulatory landscape and the challenges and opportunities in reigning in the pharmaceutical industry's influence over ADHD.

Finally, **Dr. Pecan's Wonder Elixir and the Curious Case of Overzealous Squirrels** leads us into Chapter 10, "Pursuing Independence - Strategies for Objective Research." This concluding chapter explores paths towards more independent research and unbiased information dissemination in the field of ADHD.

Throughout this book, the intertwining of anecdotal narratives with in-depth research offers a unique perspective on the influence of Big Pharma in the realm of ADHD. Each story not only humanizes the broader themes discussed in the subsequent chapters but also provides a relatable context that enhances understanding. As we journey through these pages, through the "Time for Reflection" sections, we are invited to critically examine the multifaceted relationship between pharmaceutical companies, healthcare providers, patients, and the wider public. This examination aims not just to inform but also to empower readers to navigate the complex world of ADHD with greater awareness and discernment.

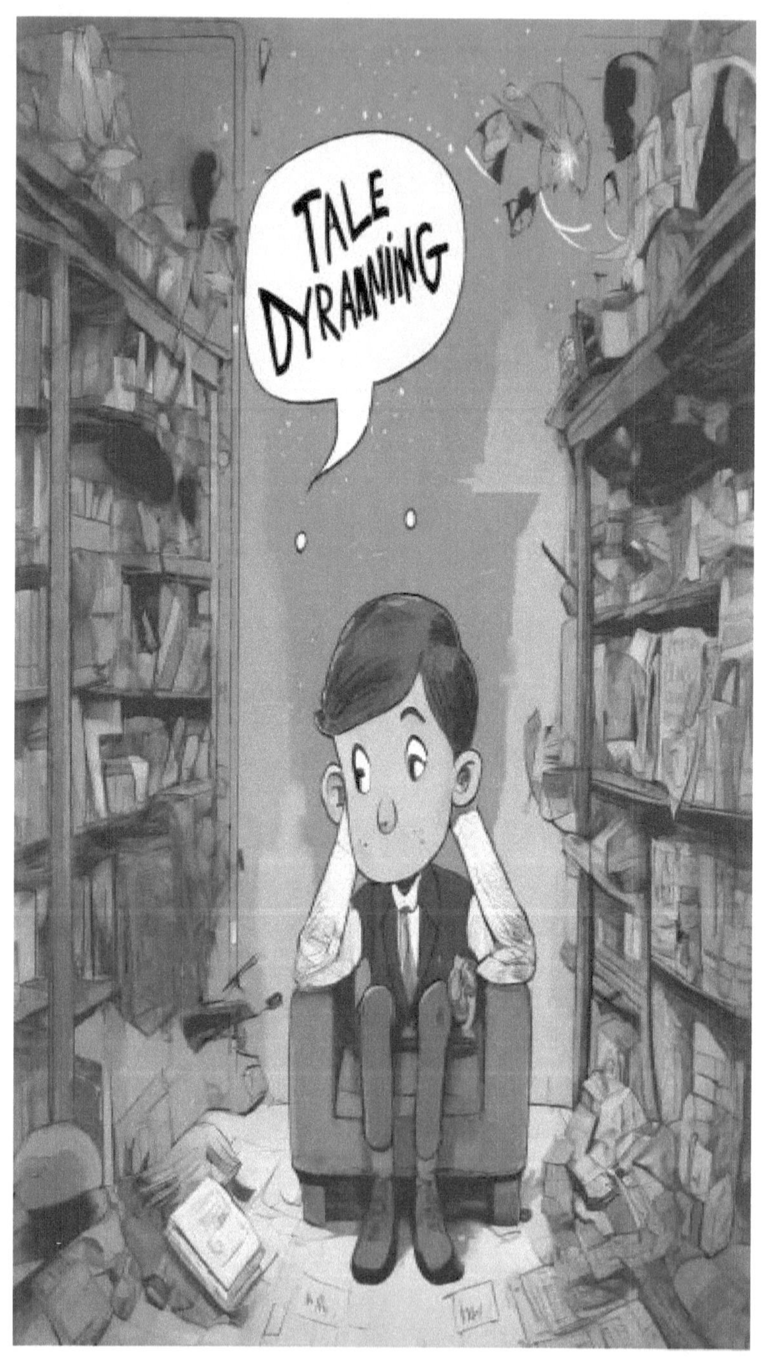
TALE
DYRANNING

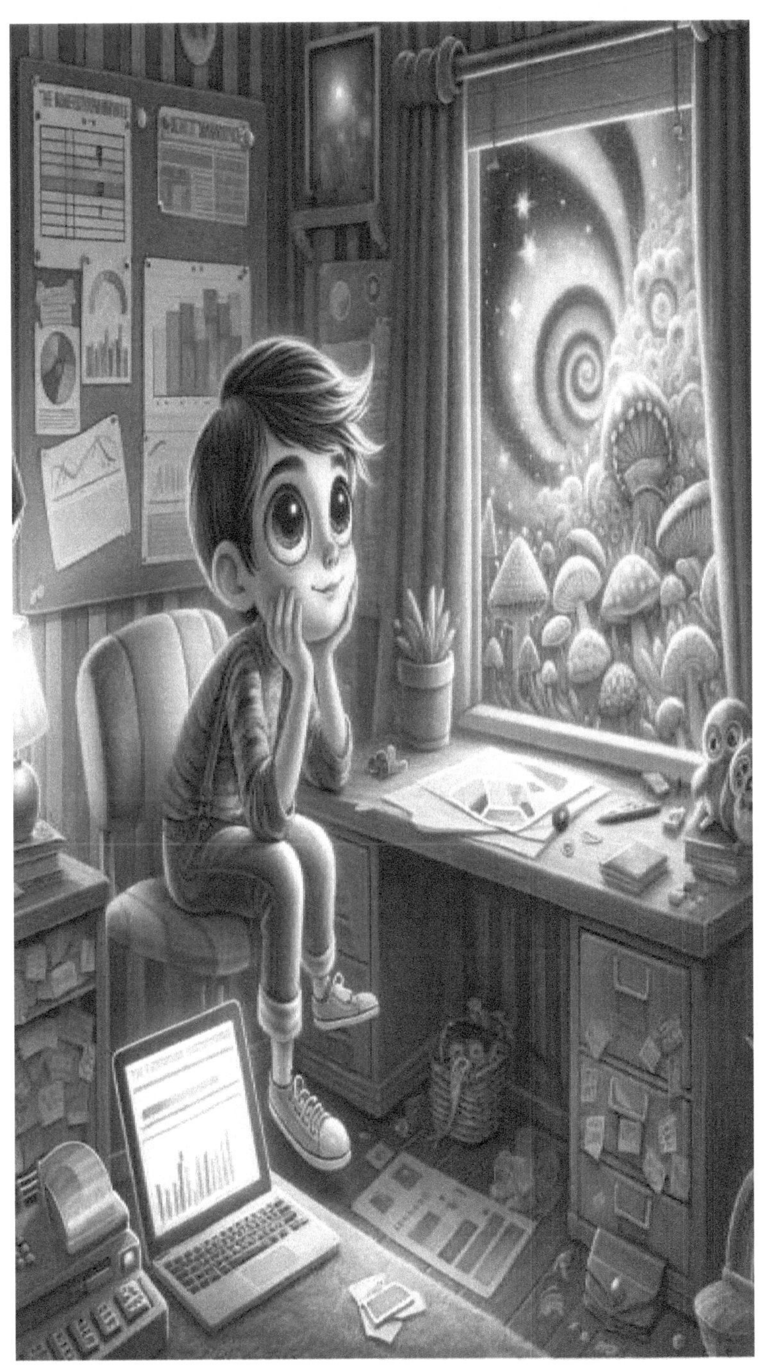

The Tale of Daydreaming Danny and the Mysterious Marketing Magicians

Danny Dover, a vivacious young boy of the tender age of 10, found solace in his imaginative world, often seen daydreaming, and getting lost in his imagination. Danny was an average, everyday preteen with not out of the ordinary, save for his tendency to lose himself in thoughts of space explorations, the mystical creatures from the Mesozoic Era – the dinosaurs, and perfecting the high wire act of swiping the last cookie from the cookie jar without drawing the sharp eyes of his elder sister. Often during school hours, Danny's teachers would catch him drifting off into his private world of imagination, particularly during the mind-numbing mathematics lectures. In Danny's view, math was a unique kind of torture that was parallel in its boredom to the act of watching paint dry.

In the midst of all these, a pharmaceutical company nicknamed "MegaPharmaCo" launched a citywide educational campaign under the title, "Are Your Kids Not Paying Attention? They Might Have ADHD!" The campaign gained attention with its colourfully designed posters that vividly caught the eye, a plethora of informational brochures replete with reasonable-sounding symptoms, and an irresistibly catchy jingle that went along the lines of, "Lost in dreams and constant stare, fret not parents, we have the pill to care!"

Having come across one such overtly persuasive ad, Danny's mother, Mrs. Dover, found herself descending into the engrossing, online world of quizzes and listicles that were specifically composed on identifying the signs of ADHD in children. Titles like "10 Signs Your Child Might Have ADHD!" seemed to be everywhere. Alarmingly, Danny seemed to exemplify around 7 out of the 10 signs outlined in these articles, which mainly revolved around rather vague definitions such as "being prone to daydreaming" and "occasional forgetfulness when it came to homework."

With the articles acting as fuel to growing concern, Mrs. Dover, intuitively feeling that something might be amiss, made up her mind to visit the renowned child psychologist in town, Dr. Knowsbest. To her great surprise, however, Dr. Knowsbest chuckled when she brought up the marketing campaign by MegaPharmaCo. He said, in a calming tone, "Ah, MegaPharmaCo. They do have a knack for crafting compelling campaigns, wouldn't you agree? But I propose we shift our focus back to Danny, and discuss him independent of any symptoms listed on a website."

Proceedings led to a detailed, comprehensive assessment taken by Dr. Knowsbest related to the overall health and behavioral traits of Danny. The result? In truth, Danny was just a perfectly average, healthy boy. His mind occasionally wandered during mathematics lessons because he perceived the subject as somewhat mundane – a sentiment shared by many, if not all of us at some point or another. Dr. Knowsbest, with his wealth of experience, suggested that a blend of interactive educational games and tutoring could serve as a potential remedy to arouse Danny's interest in the subject matter of Mathematics.

Moral of the story: For one, although Danny's propensity for daydreaming did, technically, coincide with the symptoms described by MegaPharmaCo, it is imperative to remember that any self-diagnostic list found on the internet (or enthralling jingle) is hardly comprehensive enough to paint the complete picture of a child's mental health. Validation from a professional mental health expert is still far more accurate and insightful. Secondly, as for MegaPharmaCo, their compelling marketing strategy did not end with ADHD. They moved on to launch another campaign - this time concerning the common cold. But that's a tale, delightful as it might sound, to be told on another occasion!

Chapter 1: How Big Pharma Shapes the ADHD Narrative

Attention Deficit Hyperactivity Disorder - commonly known as ADHD. Many affectionately and jokingly associate this condition with the phrase "Look, a squirrel!" as it is often equated with someone who is highly distractible. And, while it might be tempting to inject some humor into the discussion by jesting that even I, as I went about outlining this piece, had my attention wander aimlessly at least three or four times, I must attest that this is no laughing matter. (Though, of course, a quiet chuckle from time to time hardly ever hurt anyone, right?)

ADHD has increasingly seeped into everyday dialogue over the past few years, becoming a phrase regularly uttered even in non-medical contexts. This speaks volumes about our societal understanding of this neurodevelopmental condition. A memorable anecdote comes from my enchantingly eccentric next-door neighbor, Mrs. Pritchard, who earnestly proclaims that her lovable tomcat, Whiskers, must undoubtedly have ADHD as he obsessively chases his tail for hours on end. Expanded research, increased understanding, and more informed discussions around this condition have played crucial roles in improving awareness about it (even though it sometimes leads to somewhat interesting, if questionable, speculations like those of Mrs. Pritchard).

One of the most significant influences, however, can be traced back to the pharmaceutical industry. This powerful, ever-pervasive industry is often endearingly dubbed "Big Pharma" amongst individuals in the medical field, especially when they feel a bit disgruntled. Now, don't misconstrue my tone - I've attended my fair share of pharmaceutical conferences, where the appetizers alone could tempt the most resistant. This industry's wholesome influence primarily comes from initiatives like comprehensive educational campaigns, active physician outreach (sometimes involving those irresistible hors d'oeuvres), and strategic partnerships with advocacy groups. Together, these efforts contribute substantially to shaping the prevalent narrative around ADHD (Schwarz, 2013).

At the same time, it is important to note that Big Pharma's contributions aren't necessarily a negative force. They have been undeniably productive in bringing forth vital medications that effectively treat real medical conditions. However, they also have their eyes firmly fixed on a rather sizeable goal. The profits that can be derived from ADHD medication sales are tempting to say the least. For the sake of scale, consider this - in the year 2020, the global ADHD therapeutics market was valued at a staggering $11 billion! That is a sum grand enough to purchase Mrs. Pritchard's entire collection of porcelain cats, and still leave change. Projected growth for this market is substantial in the future (Transparency Market Research, 2020). With such a vast amount at stake, critics argue that

Big Pharma might sometimes cross ethical lines, potentially leading not just to increased awareness, but also fostering overdiagnoses and an unhealthy emphasis on medication (Schwartz & Cohen, 2009).

Let's take a picturesque, albeit hypothetical, trip to a small town, which we'll call 'Big Bucks, USA.' Here, it appears that ADHD diagnoses are inexplicably on the rise. What could be the possible explanation for this seemingly strange phenomenon? Research indicates that geographical regions subjected to intense marketing strategies by pharmaceutical corporations tend to report disproportionately high increases in ADHD diagnoses. Contrasting starkly with its humble neighbour 'Little Bucks,' this fictional town serves as an illustration of the power of the pharmaceutical industry (Schwarz, 2013). Albeit being beneficial in spreading awareness about ADHD, any loaded or skewed diagnostic criteria seeking mainly to advance commercial interests raise serious ethical concerns. Especially if it may lead to defining any child's daydreaming or inattentiveness as pathological solely for profit.

To wrap up, it's critical that we, as health consumers and, more importantly, as parents, siblings, friends, and individuals who may or may not personally deal with ADHD, grasp the substantial role Big Pharma plays in sculpting the ADHD narrative. In the eloquent words of my neighbour Mrs. Pritchard, "Whiskers might just be an energetic cat, not a medical case that calls for medication!" We must learn to navigate relevant information with a discerning, critical eye, sometimes even approaching it with healthy skepticism. And perhaps, we should ponder a little longer before slapping a diagnosis on the behaviour of your neighbour's pet, or even your loved ones.

Time for Reflection:

1. **Awareness and Profit Motives:** Given the interplay between raising awareness of ADHD and the financial interests of pharmaceutical companies, how do you differentiate genuine educational campaigns from those driven primarily by profit motives?

2. **Overdiagnosis Concerns:** Considering the potential influence of Big Pharma in shaping ADHD narratives, do you think it's plausible that certain behaviors or traits are now labeled as ADHD symptoms that might not have been a decade or two ago? Can you think of any examples from personal experiences or from those around you?

3. **Ethical Implications:** If a pharmaceutical company's main goal is to make a profit, where do you see the line between ethical responsibility to the patient and business interests? What would you suggest as a balance between the two?

4. **Consumer's Role:** As an informed consumer of healthcare, what steps can you take to ensure that you or your loved ones receive an accurate diagnosis and treatment

that genuinely benefits health, rather than being influenced primarily by industry-driven narratives?

References

Schwartz, S., & Cohen, S. (2009). Attention deficit hyperactivity disorder: From genes to patients. Humana Press.

Schwarz, A. (2013). The selling of attention deficit disorder. The New York Times. https://www.nytimes.com/

Transparency Market Research. (2020). Attention-Deficit/Hyperactivity Disorder (ADHD) Therapeutics Market.

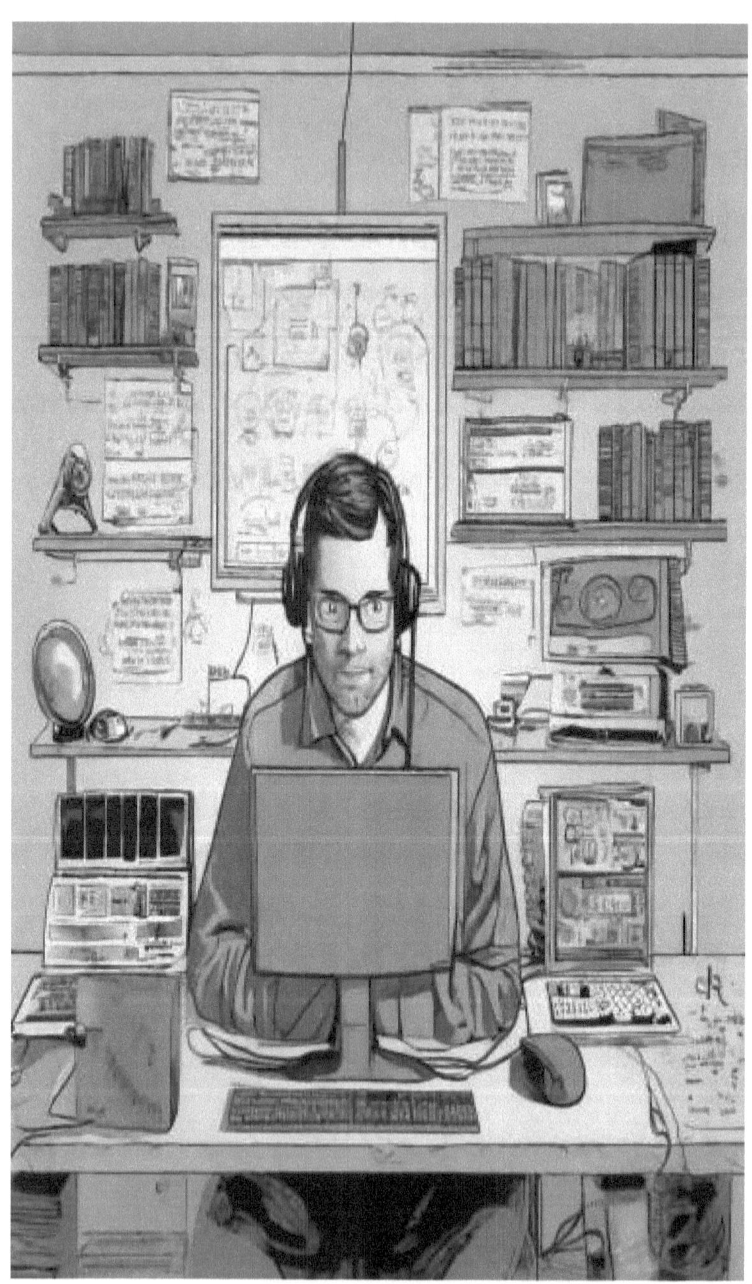

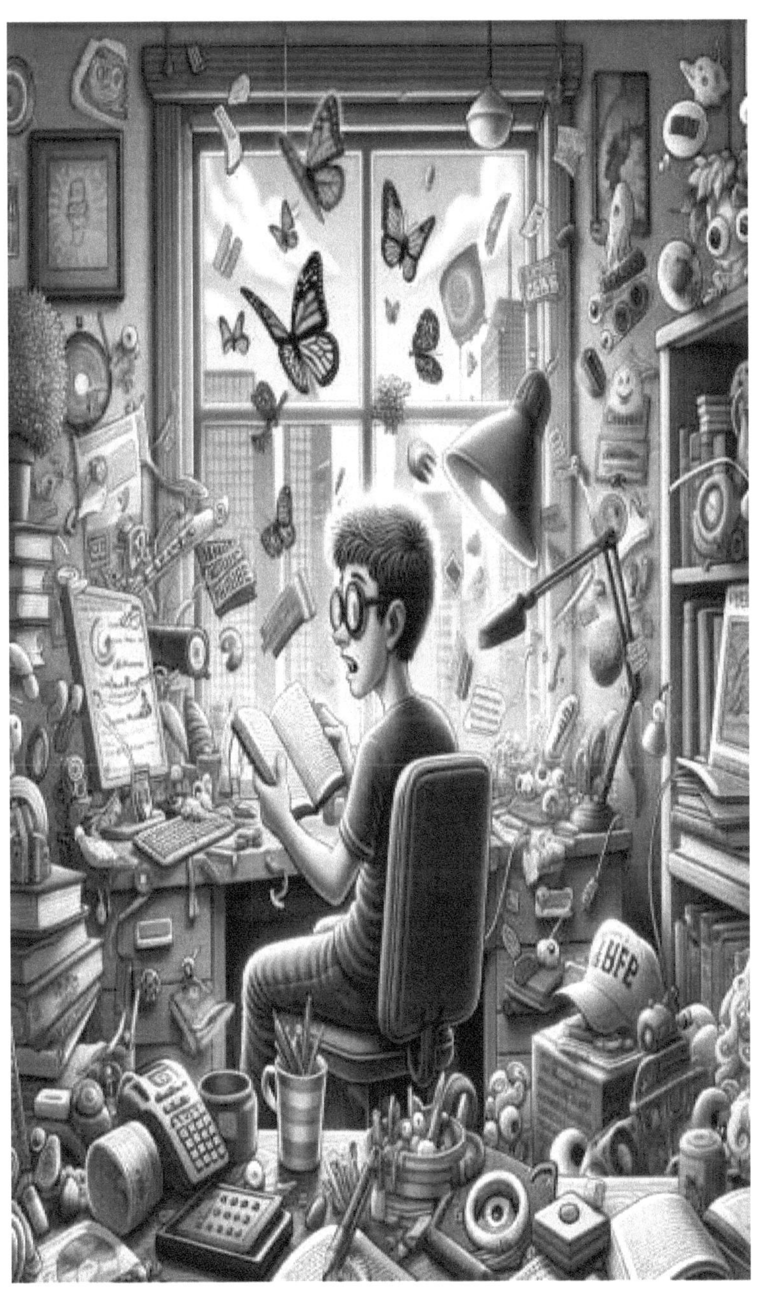

The Curious Case of Greg and the "Distract-a-lot" Syndrome

Introduction: One unsuspecting evening, Greg, an established 35-year-old software engineer, found himself engrossed in his favorite TV show during a late-night binge-watching escapade. During one of the commercial breaks, an advertisement piqued Greg's interest. The central character of this ad, uncannily reminiscent of Greg, was portrayed with a series of amusing yet typically human blunders.

Background: This advertisement met Greg's eyes during his late-night TV binge—a usual ritual for him. He saw someone, a man in the ad, who was an uncanny reflection of him. This character was portrayed with quirks that Greg immediately recognized, notably—mismatched socks—a detail so minuscule yet distinctively familiar to Greg. This man seemed to be constantly forgetting things, including his morning cup of coffee resting on the top of his car, his keys were missing twice throughout the day, and almost hilariously, he nearly mistook the salt for sugar while preparing his comforting pot of morning coffee. The creators of the advertisement then raised a profound question, potentially jolting spectators like Greg: "Could you potentially be suffering from 'Distract-a-lot' Syndrome?" This was a concern that when phrased this way, could hold the capacity to appear as more than just a harmless idiosyncrasy—it was presented as a syndrome needing rectification. The advertisement strategically concluded with a proposition of a solution— a shiny new pill named "FocusFlix."

Symptoms: Following the occurrence of this incident, Greg couldn't help but acknowledge peculiar patterns in his behavior. He found himself frequently oblivious of the location of his glasses (which, embarrassingly enough, were typically perched on the crown of his head). His concentration occasionally dwindled during official meetings. Once, in what was the cherry on top of all these incidents, he had even ventured to work sporting mis-matched shoes. This led Greg to seriously ponder on the possibility of being a passenger aboard the so-called "Distract-a-lot" Syndrome train.

Doctor visit: Disturbed by these relatable symptoms and driven by his newfound awareness, Greg sought professional help. He chose his local clinic, where he encountered Dr. Ponderosa. She was a learned professional who had conveniently just read the second chapter of a book highlighting these exact symptoms. Dr. Ponderosa couldn't help but form a wry smile upon listening to Greg's concerns. She indulged Greg in an in-depth conversation regarding his symptoms and performed a careful assessment of his habits. She made a diagnosis differing from Greg's speculation: she identified his syndrome to be not the so-called "Distract-a-lot" Syndrome, but a more contemporary and common problem— "Too-Much-Netflix-and-Not-Enough-Sleep" Disorder. Her proposed treatment was going back to basics—resting adequately, and focusing on a hobby that wasn't centered around screens.

Resolution: From this entire incident, Greg took away an invaluable lesson regarding the pervasive power of advertising and its suggestive elements. He realized that while he indeed needed to rectify his excessive screen-time and improve his sleeping habits, turning to medication to rectify every eccentric behavior or quirk was not the way to go. This incident also served as a humorous reminder to Greg to double-check his footwear before stepping out each day.

Moral of the story: The story of Greg serves to relay a critical reminder to the audience. While there may indeed be a pill to rectify a wide array of health concerns, there is non-prescribed medication to cure life's daily comical hiccups. One is wise to consult with a trusted healthcare professional to dissect the root cause of a potential problem, before jumping to any judicious conclusions potentially influenced by a carefully curated advertisement!

Chapter 2 - Big Pharma's Influence on ADHD Awareness Campaigns

Dear discerning readers, I wish to share with you an invaluable lesson gleaned from my many eventful years occupying the intriguing intersection of industry and medicine. A central axiom there is that nothing - and I mean absolutely nothing - is quite as simple or straightforward as it might initially appear. So, with your indulgence, let's embark on a fascinating excursion down the alluring, yet frequently confounding, rabbit hole of ADHD awareness campaigns and Big Pharma, shall we?

Pharmaceutical establishments often demonstrate a tremendous willingness to pour vast resources into educational outreach initiatives centered around ADHD (Attention Deficit Hyperactivity Disorder). Now, it's reasonable for you to wonder, "Why such liberal benevolence?" and "Could it be solely about fostering better understanding and awareness?" Well, in the spirit of inquisitiveness and intellectual pursuit, let's delve a bit deeper into these intriguing queries.

While these corporations make bold assertions that such "awareness campaigns" are designed with the noble and altruistic intent to assist individuals in recognizing potential symptoms, critics have expressed apprehension. They question whether such campaigns might inadvertently foster overdiagnosis through a process they've dubbed "disease-mongering," a form of fear-based marketing that revolves around broadening diagnostic boundaries (Moynihan & Cassels, 2005). Picture yourself rushing to consult your healthcare provider, utterly convinced of suffering from a severe case of "jelly belly," brought on by overindulging in an excessive quantity of sweet treats because an advertisement instilled this fear within you! Doesn't that scenario sound quite preposterous and absurd? However, these critics posit that this is essentially what is transpiring in relation to ADHD.

For instance, advertisements focused on ADHD tend to depict everyday struggles that both individuals diagnosed with the disorder and those without the condition frequently encounter, portraying these difficulties as definitive signs of ADHD. An advertisement that lingers in my memory portrayed a man who misplaces his car keys, implying this could be a symptom of ADHD. If misplaced car keys are indeed a marker for ADHD, I should be a prime candidate, having misplaced my own set of keys more than a dozen times in recent weeks. The only diagnosis I ever received for my tendency to forget is a humorous self-diagnosed condition I like to call "chronic forgetfulness," a condition, I might add, that has yet to be formally recognized in any medical literature, much to my mild annoyance. Therein lies the danger of such advertisements; they may encourage individuals to seek a medical label for behaviors and characteristics that fall within normal boundaries (Wolraich et al., 2011). These campaigns also regularly promote medication as the go-to remedy, often ignoring the potential benefits and effectiveness of alternative therapeutic avenues (Kravitz & Bell, 2007). As an individual who has managed to leave an umbrella behind on three different continents, I shudder at the thought of someone recommending a pill to cure my absent-mindedness.

It's also noteworthy that some compelling evidence suggests that these awareness campaigns tend to intensify their push as the expiration dates for drug patents loom ominously near, in a desperate bid to identify and tap into new markets (Schwarz, 2013). This strategy is somewhat akin to my beloved Aunt Mabel, who makes a point of generously distributing her infamous fruitcake as the holiday season draws to a close, thereby ensuring she has successfully cultivated a fresh, captive audience eagerly anticipating next year's batch. With diagnoses of ADHD surging in regions that are subjected to heavy advertising, the ethical implications of these campaigns become increasingly questionable. Though spreading knowledge undeniably has numerous merits, and despite Aunt Mabel's fruitcake boasting a handful of ardent fans (somewhere out there, surely!), prioritizing fiscal gains over the dissemination of balanced, objective information flirts dangerously with ethical boundaries.

As we conclude our enlightening academic sojourn, I urge you, dear readers, as discerning consumers of healthcare information, to thoughtfully ponder the underlying financial motivations behind so-called "awareness" content. Drawing on diverse expert opinions, taking a leaf out of the book of those who seek wisdom from both Aunt Mabel and Uncle Joe before settling on the perfect family potluck menu, can serve as an effective bulwark against potentially skewed marketing narratives. Informed healthcare decisions merit a discerning, comprehensive understanding rather than a knee-jerk reaction to a single persuasive marketing narrative, no matter how enthralling or festooned with tantalizing fruitcake it might appear.

Time for Reflection:

1. **Disease-Mongering and Awareness**: Considering the balance between genuine awareness campaigns and potential "disease-mongering," how can consumers differentiate between genuine health concerns and exaggerated portrayals in advertisements? Can you recall a time when an advertisement made you question or reflect on your own health?

2. **Diagnostic Boundaries**: Given the blurred lines between everyday struggles and ADHD symptoms as portrayed in ads, how do you perceive the impact of these campaigns on societal understanding of ADHD? Do you believe this

blurring is intentional, or a by-product of trying to raise awareness?

3. **Medications vs. Alternatives**: Reflect on the emphasis of medications as the primary or sole treatment option in these campaigns. How might this influence an individual's treatment choices? And, in what ways can healthcare professionals ensure patients are aware of all available treatment options?

4. **Profit vs. Genuine Concern**: Pondering on the timely push of campaigns as drug patents near expiration, how do you view the ethical implications of such marketing strategies? How can we, as consumers, ensure we're getting unbiased information and not merely being steered by profit-driven motives?

References

Kravitz, R. L., & Bell, R. A. (2007). Media, Messages, and Medication: Strategies to Reconcile What Patients Hear, What They Want, and What They Get. Journal of General Internal Medicine, 22(Suppl 2), 403-409.

Moynihan, R., & Cassels, A. (2005). Selling Sickness: How the World's Biggest Pharmaceutical Companies are Turning Us All Into Patients. Nation Books.

Schwarz, A. (2013). ADHD Nation: Children, Doctors, Big Pharma, and the Making of an American Epidemic. Scribner.

Wolraich, M. L., Wibbelsman, C. J., Brown, T. E., Evans, S. W., Gotlieb, E. M., Knight, J. R., ... & Wilens, T. (2011). Attention-Deficit/Hyperactivity Disorder Among Adolescents: A Review of the Diagnosis, Treatment, and Clinical Implications. Pediatrics, 115(6), 1734-1746.

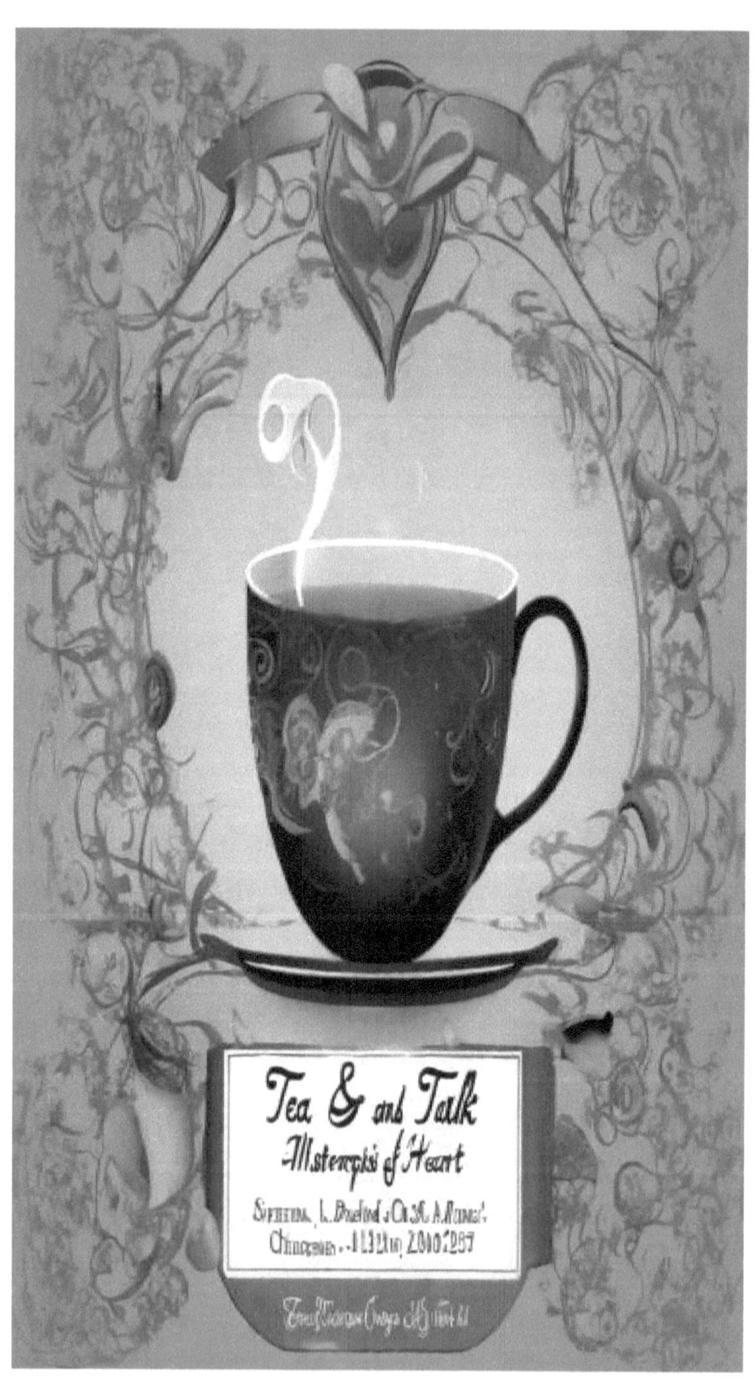

Tea & and Talk
Masterpiece of Heart

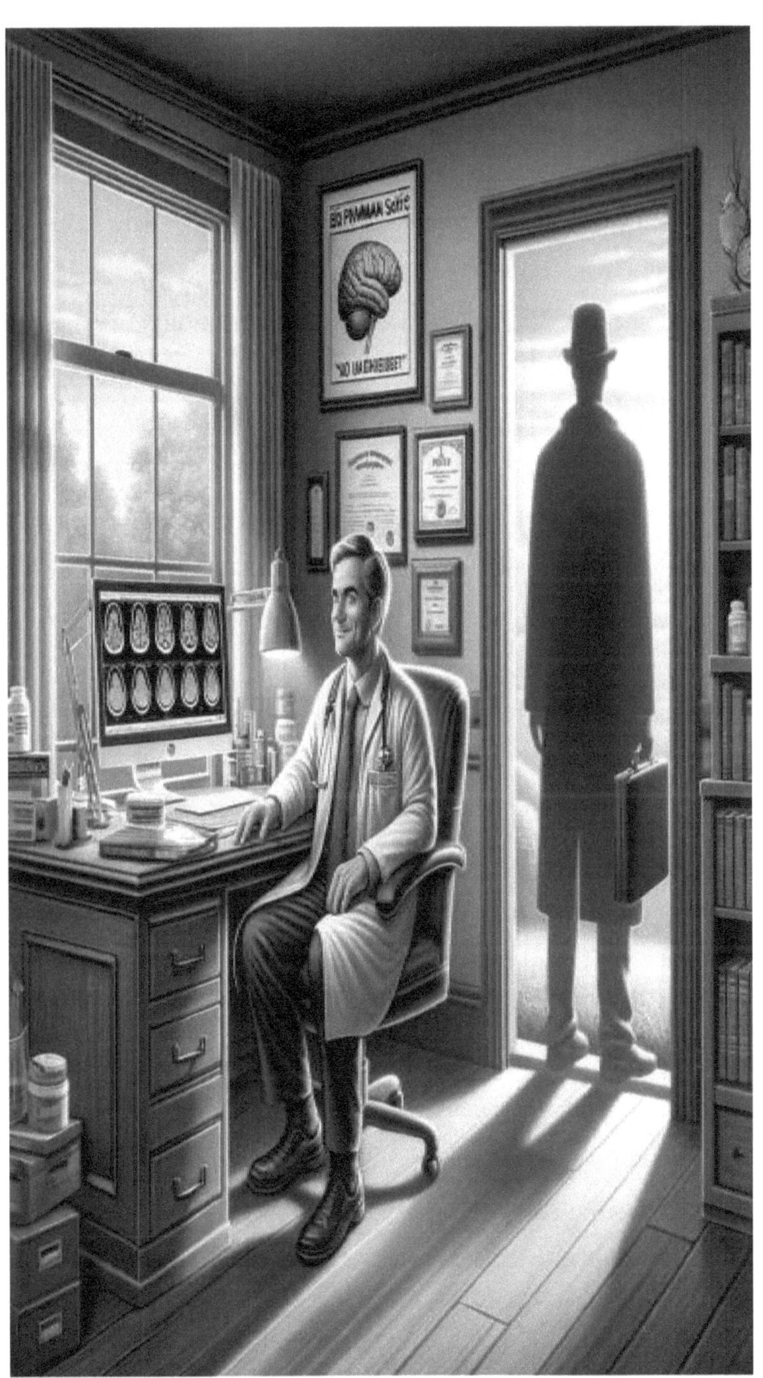

Dr. Green's "Mysterious" Change of Heart

Tucked away in the heart of the small, quaint town of Pillsville, the name that resounded in admiration through each narrow lane was Dr. Nigel Green. Fondly and widely popular as the "Tea-and-Talk" therapist, he was the local lighthouse of holistic healing. Eschewing hasty pharmaceutical prescriptions, Dr. Green extended a cozy ambience, a steaming cuppa tea, and the promise of a heartfelt conversation that often proved therapeutic in itself to his patients. His firm belief in the power of herbal remedies resulted in him indirectly becoming the benefactor behind the prospering local tea shops who saw a considerable increase in their business, thanks to Dr. Green's unshakeable faith in the healing powers of herbal tea over chemical laden pills.

This tranquil routine of Pillsville was suddenly disrupted one seemingly ordinary morning. Mr. Cashmore, a sharply dressed pharmaceutical representative from the giant corporation, Big MedCorp, confidently strode into Dr. Green's traditionally set office. He came bearing exciting gifts: a suitcase jam-packed with glossy, attention-grabbing brochures, pens branded with intimidating medication names, and, the cherry on top, a state-of-the-art coffee machine. He humorously suggested the machine was necessary "For those demanding days when even a soothing cup of tea just doesn't cut it." Flashing his most charming grin, he winked.

In the wake of this corporate invasion, the cherished "Tea-and-Talk" sessions tragically morphed into the cold, impersonal "Pills-and-Pamphlets" appointments. One such instance was Ms. Jenkins, a kind lady who had often sought Dr. Green's advice about her mild insomnia and found solace in his recommendation of chamomile tea. She now found herself handed a slick pamphlet titled "ZzZleepify," peddled as the latest heralding sensation in the world of sleep pills.

This sudden shift in Dr. Green's approach prompted uneasy whispers to ripple through the townsfolk. Mrs. Thompson, who was fond of cats, recounted an incident, "Once, when I was feeling rather down because my beloved cat Whiskers had disappeared, before I knew it, Dr. Green was pushing 'MoodLift Max' pills towards me. Just last week, he'd have distracted me with cute pictures of his kittens to cheer me up."

Then came the climactic moment that resulted in the metaphorical alarm bells ringing across Pillsville. Young Timmy, a rather anxious student who'd perennially been advised by Dr. Green to practice deep breathing exercises to combat his school anxieties, was suddenly handed a glossy booklet promoting "CalmKidz" medication. With the innocence and candor typical of an 8-year-old, he braved a query, "But Dr. Green, isn't this the controversial stuff that television advertisements peddle in between my favorite Saturday morning cartoons?"

The undercurrent of dissent rose to a roar, word spread like wildfire, and soon, a town meeting was hastily scheduled. Cornered by a throng of concerned, caffeine-deprived townspeople, Dr. Green finally admitted, "Okay, okay! Perhaps I let myself get a bit carried away with the allure of the ultra-modern coffee machine and the persuasive demos Mr. Cashmore had so enthusiastically presented."

And, as swiftly as the invasion had occurred, the unsettling coffee machine was discarded, making way for a fresh assortment of aromatic teas and pleasant conversation. Pillsville finally regained its old serene charm, although there conjecture persists that Dr. Green occasionally indulges in a sneaky cup of coffee. However, this clandestine deviation is merely tolerated, as long as it's accompanied by a hearty, good old chat.

Moral of the story: Despite the glimmering appeal of a shiny new coffee machine, it could never truly replace the authenticity of heartfelt patient care. Adding to this, one could always count on the blissful honesty of an 8-year-old to highlight the elephant in the room!

Chapter 3 - Pharma and the Medicalization of ADHD

Upon reading this, I would cordially invite you to pop that tab off your favorite can of soda, or, if you prefer a more calming experience, prepare a soothing cup of chamomile tea. Comfortably nestled where you are, let's take a deep dive into the in-depth details of Big Pharma and its expansive reach—a reach that sometimes results in peculiar situations that are sure to raise an eyebrow or two. It's as if you had a charming cousin, let's call him Big Cousin, who unfailingly found a way to turn every family gathering into a grand display of their own importance. Now, imagine, if you will, that Big Cousin was not just a member of your family but an influential pharmaceutical company. This is the awe-inspiring, and sometimes dubious, reach of Big Pharma.

The sphere of influence of Big Pharma is vast and extends far beyond the basic realm of advertising. It delves deep into the interweaving relationships with healthcare providers, even from the most granular sectors of the healthcare industry. A common perception that many have, from the outside looking in, is that these drug firms mainly aim, with a purpose as noble as a knight from an age-old age, to educate the medical fraternity. Ah, such an idealistic and admirable intention, you might think. However, wait just a moment, because there is a particularly troubling plot twist. Financial ties with physicians, ambiguously ethical and valid as they may be, raise substantial concerns over their ethical implications (Ornstein & Weber, 2016). The analogy here may seem outlandish, but bear with me. It's somewhat like inviting Big Cousin to your extravagant wedding, despite their narcissistic tendencies, primarily because they have promised to gift you something grand and lavish. And then, as you excitedly tear open the gift-wrapped box, you discover, much to your dismay, that it's a blender. Again.

Interactions induced by Big Pharma, often in the form of sponsored education, have the power to shape the perspectives of healthcare providers. Picture a scene, and no, not Sicily in 1985 (I apologize, that's a 'Golden Girls' reference—perhaps I've watched a bit too much of that show). Let's instead visualize a plush, cozy conference room. Here, industry experts passionately expound on the marvels of new drugs. You're served shiny, polished pamphlets on a platter, seated on cushy reclining chairs, even offered sandwiches—probably tuna with a side of dill pickle. However, multiple research studies— and these are consistent in their findings—concur that such industry-funded events tend to emphasize the benefits of pharmaceutical drugs while dramatically downplaying or entirely overlooking alternatives that exist (Fickweiler et al., 2017). It feels akin to stepping into a grand buffet, filled with a variety of mouth-watering dishes, yet being told the only delicacy worth trying is the mashed potatoes. Simultaneously, these gatherings tend to cultivate a breed of providers who grow inclined to prescribe precisely those drugs that were highlighted during the event, regardless of their efficacy or necessity (Sah & Fugh-Berman, 2013). If I, the narrator of this tale, were to receive a nickel for every time I've seen this happen, I'd probably be swimming in a sea of nickels.

Big Pharma, staying true to its infamous reputation for extensive influence, molds the conversations that take place between patients and clinicians through physician detailing, or to explain it in simpler terms, drop-in visits to medical practitioners by drug representatives to promote specific medications. It's a bit like those pesky door-to-door salespeople we've all come across, except here, they're knocking on your doctor's office door instead of yours. While admittedly informative, these interactions often incentivize spending on promotional materials of their products, which are often exaggerated sales pitches, rather than clinically instructive materials (Dana & Loewenstein, 2003). To put it into layman's terms, it's akin to getting a colorful, glossy pamphlet on the wonders of a vacuum cleaner, written with such fervor that you're convinced it's an absolute necessity for your home. Still, the pamphlet conveniently forgets to mention that it might cause a short circuit if used simultaneously with other appliances.

Critics of Big Pharma argue its tactics risk a dangerous consequence—pathologizing conditions to fit the narrative of the drugs they market rather than objectively diagnosing disorders

(Angell, 2004). In other words, it's like trying to fit a square peg into a round hole and insisting, with unwavering confidence, that it's the latest design trend to take the world by storm. This risk is particularly relevant in psychiatry, where the clear definition of symptoms often blur into each other. Here, the sway of Big Pharma could potentially mean over-medicalizing issues that could be addressed more wholesomely through a holistic approach (Moynihan & Cassels, 2005). One instance that resonates strongly with this issue is a rather humorous anecdote about a colleague, Dr. Roberts. He once had a patient who claimed to have self-diagnosed himself with "Chocolate-induced Acute Joy Syndrome," after attending a seminar on food addictions sponsored, of course, by Big Pharma. This unexpected claim served as a gentle reminder, even amidst the humor, of the potential hazards of over-medicalization.

To ensure patient-centered care, clinicians should diligently scrutinize all forms of messaging coming from pharmaceutical companies, ensuring they aren't swept away by potential biases, however subtle they may be. Instead, they should seek the tricky but necessary balance through guidelines that emphasize comprehensive evaluation and care. It's similar to the process of sieving flour while baking. You want to get rid of the lumps (or in this case, misleading pharmaceutical propaganda) and keep the pure, essential elements of care. Informed consent, a cornerstone of any healthcare decision, necessitates a clear understanding of how financial ties sometimes lead medical practitioners to privilege commercial priorities over medical ones. Close on the heels of our earlier familial analogy, don't forget that just because Big Cousin dangles a tempting blender—a shiny piece of kitchen equipment you may have coveted for long— that doesn't mean it's the right fit for your kitchen or, extending the analogy, your health. With that thought-provoking note, here's a toast to a future where healthcare decisions prioritize patient wellbeing over commercial interests. Cheers!

Time for Reflection:

1. **Pharmaceutical Influence:** Reflecting on personal experiences or those of close ones, can you recall instances where medication was prescribed may have been influenced more by pharmaceutical promotion rather than an objective evaluation of the patient's needs? How did that make you feel about the integrity of the medical profession?

2. **Pharma-sponsored Education:** Have you ever attended or been aware of a medical seminar or conference sponsored by a pharmaceutical company? If so, were you able to discern biases in the information presented, favoring the company's products? How might this skew the perceptions of healthcare providers?

3. **Patient-Clinician Dialog:** Thinking about past doctor visits, were there moments when the doctor seemed particularly keen on prescribing a specific medication without providing ample alternatives or holistic remedies?

Could pharma influence have played a role, and how would you approach such situations differently in the future?

4. **Medicalization vs. Holistic Approaches:** Considering the potential for conditions to be pathologized to fit certain medications, have you ever wondered if a diagnosis you or someone you know received was overly reliant on medication solutions? How might a balance between holistic and medication-focused care be achieved in such scenarios?

References

Angell, M. (2004). The truth about the drug companies: How they deceive us and what to do about it. Random House.

Dana, J., & Loewenstein, G. (2003). A social science perspective on gifts to physicians from industry. JAMA, 290(2), 252-255.

Fickweiler, F., Fickweiler, W., & Urbach, E. (2017). Interactions between physicians and the pharmaceutical industry generally and sales representatives specifically and their association with physicians' attitudes and prescribing habits: a systematic review. PLOS Medicine, 14(9), e1002361.

Moynihan, R., & Cassels, A. (2005). Selling Sickness: How the World's Biggest Pharmaceutical Companies are Turning Us All Into Patients. Nation Books.

Ornstein, C., & Weber, T. (2016). How pharma sales reps help me be a more up-to-date doctor. Health Affairs. https://www.healthaffairs.org/

Sah, S., & Fugh-Berman, A. (2013). Physicians under the influence: Social psychology and industry marketing strategies. The Journal of Law, Medicine & Ethics, 41(3), 665-672.

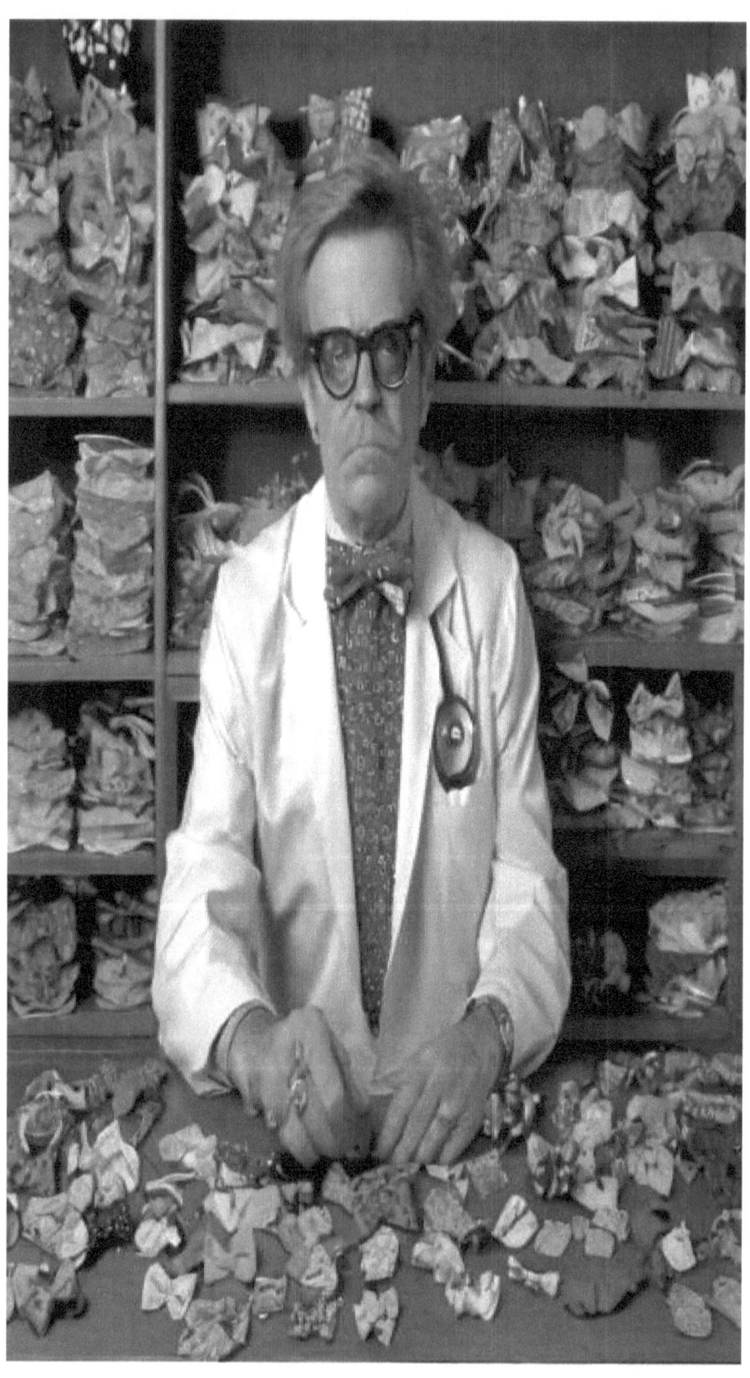

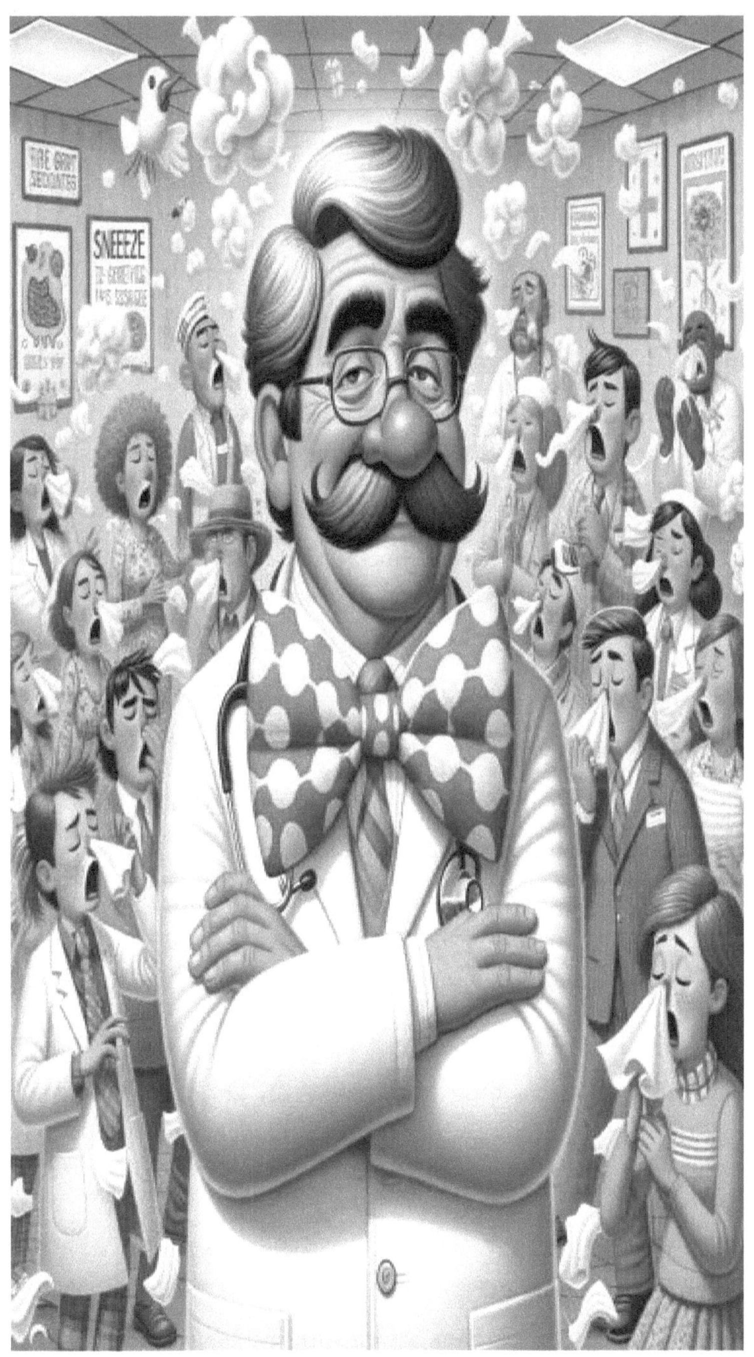
SNEEZE

Dr. Larry and the Great "Sneezitis" Epidemic

Dr. Larry was an eccentric, flamboyant psychiatrist who was widely known for his whimsical and vibrant bow tie collection. His career was characterized by a constant thirst for discovery and exploration. His eccentricities, however, didn't stop him from being highly respected in his field. One ordinary day, he stumbled upon what he fervently believed was a groundbreaking discovery—something that he couldn't wait to share with the world. He coined it "Sneezitis," a novel condition that was characterized by sporadic, uncontrollable sneezing triggered solely by the mere thought of pepper.

Coincidentally, Dr. Larry enjoyed a close association with Big Pepper Pharma. This company stood notable for being the world's largest and most influential pepper exporter, supplier, and distributor. This relationship seemed so seamless that it was considered primarily beneficial in nature, often underestimated in any potentially negative aspects.

Upon hearing of this intriguing discovery by Dr. Larry, Big Pepper Pharma had become extraordinarily enthralled. The idea sparked their interest and held promise in terms of capitalization --an opportunity they were quick to capture. Big Pepper Pharma therefore committed to robustly backing up the "Sneezitis" theory, fervently funding extensive research with the aim of solidifying the legitimacy of "Sneezitis" as a bona fide medical condition. Quite conveniently, they also found themselves developing an anti-sneezing nasal spray, presumably a 'remedy' for this spontaneous piperine-allergic sneezing.

Dr. Larry, equipped with this invaluable support, worked relentlessly, aiming to have the "Sneezitis" included in the Diagnostic and Statistical Manual of Mental Disorders (DSM). His proposal was pretty intense—made with the aspiration of gaining recognition in psychiatry.

With time, following a thorough examination series supported mainly by Big Pepper Pharma, studies began emerging—one after another. These studies confirmed the existence of Sneezitis, emphasizing its rampant prevalence worldwide. Suddenly, it seemed like everyone, every unassuming person you looked at, was showing signs, winning prescriptions of the anti-sneezing nasal spray; the figures were skyrocketing.

Local establishments, especially small-scale diners, abruptly chose to remove pepper from their tables altogether. All for the fear of provoking or triggering a Sneezitis episode, some controversial decision that generated mixed reactions from patrons—bemused, bewildered, and somewhat skeptical, especially pepper-lovers.

Nonetheless, a section of independent researchers—those without any vested interests in Big Pepper Pharma or any seasoning conglomerate—had their reservations about this. Their skepticism was piqued as they reviewed the findings, and they started posing questions. Their analysis suggested that perhaps the act of sneezing at merely the thought of pepper was nothing more than a natural response—not an ailment demanding treatment.

As public awareness increased, debates and discussions about the epidemic of Sneezitis became widespread. Questions surrounding the ethics of Big Pepper Pharma's influence rose to the surface. Is it possible that Big Pepper Pharma exaggerated a condition—Illness inflation—to boost the sales of their new anti-sneezing nasal spray? While it's an interrogative we can't confidently answer, one vivid fact made itself clear—Dr. Larry's bow ties became even more colorful, more vibrant following this discovery. Word around the corridors was that these snazzy bow ties were generous gifts from Big Pepper Pharma's latest line of fashionable accessories—an interesting coincidence, one might say.

Takeaway. Balancing between potential conflicts of interest and actual medical development can sometimes seem as convoluted as deciding whether or not to pepper your pasta. It's a constant reminder that we need to exercise discretion with caution and ensure guidelines prioritize overall well-being over fanciful diagnoses—an ounce of prevention is worth a pound of cure, after all. Healthcare is about wellness, not business.

Chapter 4: Shaping the Definition - Big Pharma's Influence on Diagnostic Criteria

Ah, the Diagnostic and Statistical Manual of Mental Disorders, colloquially referred to as the DSM, a significant publication circulated by the influential American Psychiatric Association. Its reputation precedes it; it's somewhat analogous to the "Who's Who" catalogue, specifically but not exclusive to the realm of mental health disorders. Much like a celebrity list, it includes a collection of defined disorders, causing frequent discussions and debates regarding who gets included, and conversely, who is left out. A focal point of that discourse often orbits around a colossal disorder, better known as ADHD, an acronym for Attention Deficit Hyperactivity Disorder.

Critics have often made comparisons that liken the relationship existing between the DSM and the powerful pharmaceutical sector, or "Big Pharma," to that of a teenager with their first love. It's as if a certain infatuation exists, leading to the DSM potentially being influenced much more profoundly they might care to openly acknowledge.

Indeed, it's almost beyond question that the DSM serves a pivotal function in the definition and recognition of disorders such as ADHD. Nevertheless, a certain raft of naysayers put forward the proposition that Big Pharma has been perhaps surreptitiously writing sweet, persuasive nothings in the DSM's yearbook, metaphorically speaking, of course. A somewhat revelatory study published in 2013 by PLOS Medicine disclosed that more than half of the members comprising the DSM-5 task force were reporting some form of industry associations, such as being in receipt of research funding (Cosgrove et al., 2014).

A personal recollection comes to mind from a professional acquaintance of mine, who shared a humorous observation. He humorously quipped that he could utilise a dime for each instance a pharmaceutical company made attempts to build a rapport with him at a conference, he would have amassed enough to independently finance his own investigative research. Such a comment might be dismissed as a jest, but as adages often state, there exists a kernel of truth in each joke.

Scientific research and investigations conducted subsequently have somewhat failed to assuage these concerns. In reality, they could even be seen as adding additional fuel to the debate's fire. One notable review discovered that studies generously funded by drug companies displayed an uncanny propensity for generating results that fortuitously favored their benefactors' products, particularly when compared to unaffiliated, independent research (Lundh et al., 2017). It should stand to reason that as diagnostic criteria expands, so too does the market; thus more "patients" would logically lead to an uplift in the rates of prescriptions. Consider the analogy of casting a wider net leading to capturing more fish. However, in this metaphorical circumstance, the fish we're discussing are being prescribed medication.

Critics strongly pose that there's something a bit suspicious, akin to discovering your canine companion sitting adjacent to a toppled trash can with garbage chaotically scattered everywhere, though insisting his innocence. While we can't unequivocally prove that financial motivations play puppeteer behind the scenes, the mere suggestion or perception of these conflicts can cast an uncomfortable shadow on the integrity of the guidelines. It's eerily comparable to that one relative who cannot resist sharing embarrassing anecdotes at family gatherings; regardless of their authenticity, these stories influence perceptions.

To ensure that medical guidelines are not unduly swayed by the mellifluous serenades of Big Pharma, implementing recusals for significant industry affiliations can be perceived as a worthy step moving forward. It emphasizes the necessity of maintaining balanced care, giving superior preference over commercial priorities. This is vitally important because, at the conclusion of each day, patients should not be ensnared in an ugly tug-of-war between corporate profit and the delivery of proper, ethical care.

Time for Reflection:

1. **Influence and Objectivity:** Reflect on a time in your life when you felt influenced or swayed by external factors, especially when there was a potential gain involved. How does this personal experience shape your understanding of the possible influences Big Pharma might have on the DSM task force members?

2. **Broadening Criteria and Implications:** Given that broadened diagnostic criteria can lead to more prescriptions, how do you perceive the balance between ensuring that individuals receive the care they need versus the risk of over-diagnosis and potential over-medication?

3. **Trust and Transparency:** How important is it to you that medical guidelines are free from potential conflicts of interest? Do you believe full transparency about financial ties would restore trust, or is it more about the actions taken (like recusals) that would rebuild confidence in the system?

4. **Patient-Centered Care:** Drawing from the last point in the chapter, how would you prioritize patient care in a system where commercial priorities are inescapable? How can we ensure that patient well-being remains at the forefront of diagnosis and treatment, even when commercial interests are at play?

References:

Cosgrove, L., Bursztajn, H. J., Erlich, D. R., Wheeler, E. E., & Shaughnessy, A. F. (2014). Conflicts of interest and the quality of recommendations in clinical guidelines. Journal of Evaluation in Clinical Practice, 20(6), 674-681.

Lundh, A., Lexchin, J., Mintzes, B., Schroll, J. B., & Bero, L. (2017). Industry sponsorship and research outcome. Cochrane Database of Systematic Reviews, 2.

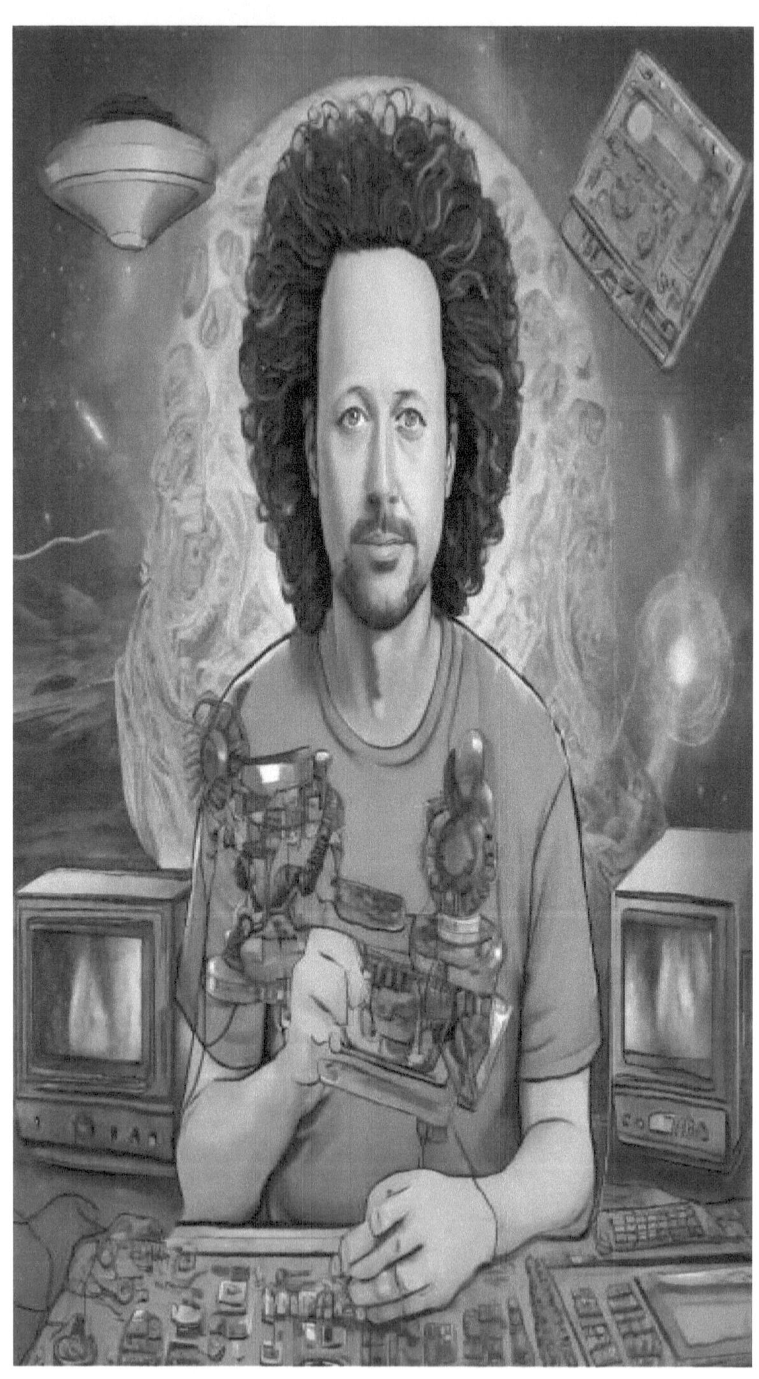

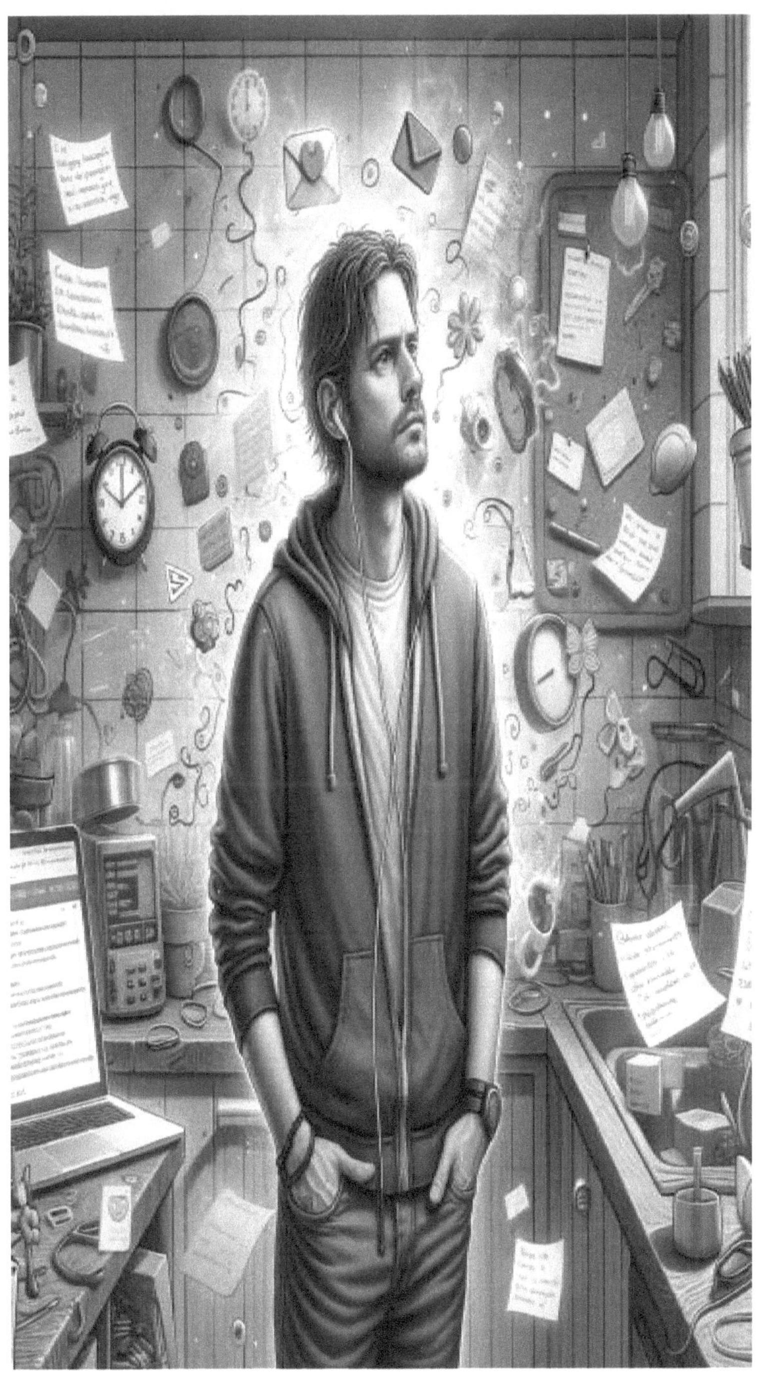

Tim's *Enlightening* Journey to the "Chronic
Distraction Disorder" Diagnosis

In the lively development hub of the city, a spry, agile, 35-year-old software developer named Tim was fully absorbed in enjoying his usual weekly indulgence in a thrilling "Ancient Aliens" marathon viewing session. Amidst this engrossing visual journey into the unknown, Tim was captivated by a slick, polished advertisement that suddenly interrupted his extraterrestrial binge watching.

Set against the soothing and emotional background of soft, melodic piano music, a seasoned, professional-looking actor with a commanding presence introduced viewers to the concept of "Chronic Distraction Disorder (CDD)"— a condition that until then, Tim had not known about. The actor, with his expertly-staged, wistful expressions, perfectly encapsulated the symptoms of the condition. He gazed longingly at a delicate, mesmerizing butterfly, got hopelessly lost while performing the simple morning ritual of pouring coffee, and even appeared deeply introspective and immensely contemplative over the seemingly mundane incident of his breakfast toast popping up.

This seemingly ordinary, everyday struggle struck a chord with Tim. He distinctly remembered one recent incident where he wandered purposelessly into the kitchen, completely forgetting his initial intention of making toast. A moment of realization struck him, forcing him to exclaim aloud, "That's me! Just last week, I forgot why I walked into the kitchen. It was for toast!" He felt a sudden camaraderie with the actor depicting the condition and an understanding of what he was going through.

Engaging further in self-introspection, Tim started identifying more unnoticed symptoms which now felt glaringly obvious. There was the unforgettable instance when he misplaced his glasses despite them resting on his head, or when he found himself lost in thought wondering curiously about his pet cat's possible belief in aliens. The evidence was clear - or at least, it seemed clear to Tim. He felt a rush of self-affirmation and validation, exclaiming, "CDD! I must have it!"

Excitedly, he decided to visit his doctor. Tim's doctor was Dr. Nancy Wiseowl, a seasoned, pragmatic clinician with an unwavering respect for evidence-based medical practices and a peculiar penchant for wearing distinct owl-themed brooches. Upon hearing Tim's self-diagnosis, Dr. Wiseowl responded, gently concealing her amusement, "Ah yes, Chronic Distraction Disorder – I believe I read about it in the 'Journal of Imaginary Ailments' between 'Uncontrollable Pinky Twitches' and 'Sudden Cravings for Moon Cheese'."

As laughter echoed in the room, the doctor-patient duo then engaged in a thoughtful, genuine conversation about Tim's experiences and anxieties. In her usual calm, empathetic manner, Dr. Wiseowl explained to Tim how sometimes, advertisements could cherry-pick information or oversimplify complex medical conditions. They delved into potential holistic approaches to mitigate his occasional forgetfulness, which when combined with tried and tested, evidence-based methods, could be a practical way to alleviate his concerns.

In the concluding moments of their conversation, Tim left the clinic not with a prescription for the CDD "miracle drug" as seen on TV, but with a renewed and profound understanding of himself. He was determined to view the next attractive, glitzy advertisement with a more critical eye, questioning the narratives packaged so appealingly. Dr. Wiseowl could congratulate herself for another instance where she had navigated the murky waters of direct-to-consumer influenced diagnoses thoroughly and efficiently, adding another metaphorical feather to her cap—or to put it more appropriately, to her owl-themed brooch collection.

Chapter 5: Selling Sickness - The Risks of DTC Advertising

Alas, the age of Direct-to-consumer (DTC) campaigns! I'm sure you resonate with me when I say there was a time, not so long ago, when we could settle down to stream our favorite TV or internet show and not be besieged by an endless barrage of commercials. Do you recall the ubiquitous advertisements featuring tranquil, contented people frolicking in glittering fields, the implication being that a miraculous pill had wiped away all their troubles? Those were the good old days. Today, DTC campaigns often blur and distort the typically clear-cut relationships between symptoms and drugs. They suggest insidiously that if you've ever felt a tad unfocused while, for example, mulling over the age-old conundrum of whether the chicken or the egg made its appearance first, you might well be a candidate for medication. It's alarming how these campaigns normalize even the slightest struggles as being seemingly credentialled for medication.

In a scenario reminiscent of an intricate detective series plot twist, the influence of advertising inflated prodigiously in the aftermath of the 1997 deregulation party. And lo and behold, ADHD diagnoses experienced a surge eerily similar to the way yeast balloons in home-bread-making experiments gone awry, as cited by Ventola (2011). One cannot help but ponder whether Sherlock Holmes would announce with his trademark flourish, "The game is afoot!" or perhaps amend it to, "The ad is afoot!" The perils become dauntingly evident when it is the luring, seductive call of marketing, rather than the sagely, owl-like acumen of clinical judgment, which steers unsuspecting patients into clinics.

There's something about advertisements that endows them with a unique ability for dumbing down the complexities of human health, akin to transforming a Picasso masterpiece to a simplistic paint-by-numbers portrait. They tend to oversimplify multifaceted conditions much like an overzealous fan attempting to squeeze all seven riveting seasons of Game of Thrones into a single, pithy tweet. Their primary enticement usually orbits around managing those troublesome individual symptoms, while conveniently sidelining the all-encompassing ballet of holistic wellness as underscored by Bell et al. (2010). And it would be remiss to overlook our quiet champions— the non-pharmaceutical therapies. Much like the understated pupil at the back of the class who happens to be a whizz at cracking complicated problems, these potentially life-changing treatments often remain shadowed. This unfortunate circumstance persists despite their well-documented efficacy, particularly when they dutifully collaborate with conventional medications to perform synergistically– a dynamic duo of effectiveness, according to Wolraich et al. (2019).

Let's journey back in time to a rather enlightening weekend when I decided to play detective (or in other words, indulge in intensive research while savoring a hot cup of tea). A penetrating analysis by Public Citizen unearthed something quite startling. Regions subjected to the undiluted power of DTC ad campaigns bore witness to an unprecedented increase in diagnoses, compared to their more sedate neighbors, as observed by Baumgartner et al. (2014). Of course, I'd be the last person to leap to conclusions – after all, in my more naive days, I sincerely believed socks vanished from the washing machine due to a nefarious sock-gorging monster. Nevertheless, it's a nagging, tough-to-dismiss feeling that this aggressive promotion may be more focused on inflating markets rather than improving public health conditions.

And here's a jaw-dropping fact: empirical evidence embedded in rigorous scientific studies suggests that the purported benefits of DTC campaigns are minimal at best, opening up a Pandora's box of unforeseen risks and side effects. Until we can secure robust, unassailable research that incontrovertibly affirms the authenticity and utility of these ads, and ensures they portray the comprehensive picture of human health (akin to painting the full Mona Lisa and not merely her alluring smile), adopting a balanced, judicious approach seems prudent. Drawing from my decades of experience, I strongly believe that regulatory measures should prioritize the sage advice of seasoned, stethoscope-brandishing healthcare providers, rather than the profit-seeking jingle of catchy commercials. At the twilight of every day, patients undoubtedly deserve comprehensive treatment plans meticulously crafted by medical virtuosi, not scripts artfully penned by industry copywriters.

Time for Reflection:

1. **Symptom-Drug Connections**: Reflect on the advertisements you have seen recently. Can you identify instances where DTC campaigns seemed to blur the lines between everyday struggles and medical conditions? How did those ads make you feel about your own experiences or the experiences of those around you?

2. **Holistic Well-being vs. Discrete Symptoms**: Think about the broader picture of health and well-being. How might a focus on individual symptoms, as portrayed in many ads, detract from understanding and addressing the root causes or interconnected issues in mental and physical health?

3. **Influence of Intensive Advertising**: Considering the link between regions with intensive DTC ads and a rise in diagnoses, how do you think advertising shapes societal perceptions of certain conditions or diseases? Have you or someone you know ever felt compelled to seek a diagnosis or treatment due to an advertisement?

4. **Medical Expertise vs. Industry Narratives**: Reflect on the balance between patient empowerment and the influence of external narratives. How can individuals ensure that their healthcare decisions are primarily informed by medical expertise and personal needs rather than industry-driven messaging?

References:

Baumgartner, J. C., Wolfe, J. L., Casaneuva, C., DiPietro, N. A., Henry, N. J., Kaufman, M., ... & Person, S. D. (2014). Expansion of pediatric diagnoses and stimulant prescription rates in commercially insured young children. Journal of Child and Adolescent Psychopharmacology, 24(10), 579-584.

Bell, L., Long, S., Garvan, C., & Bussing, R. (2010). The impact of teacher credentials on ADHD stigma perceptions. Psychology in the Schools, 48(2), 184-197.

Ventola, C. L. (2011). Direct-to-consumer pharmaceutical advertising: Therapeutic or toxic? Pharmacy and Therapeutics, 36(10), 669-674.

Wolraich, M., Wierzbicki, G., Bax, A.L., Bubba, J., Chavez, S.R., Craft, J., ... & Kryzer, E. (2019). Management of children with ADHD: A multi-stakeholder

perspective. Journal of Attention Disorders, 23(14),
1651-1668.

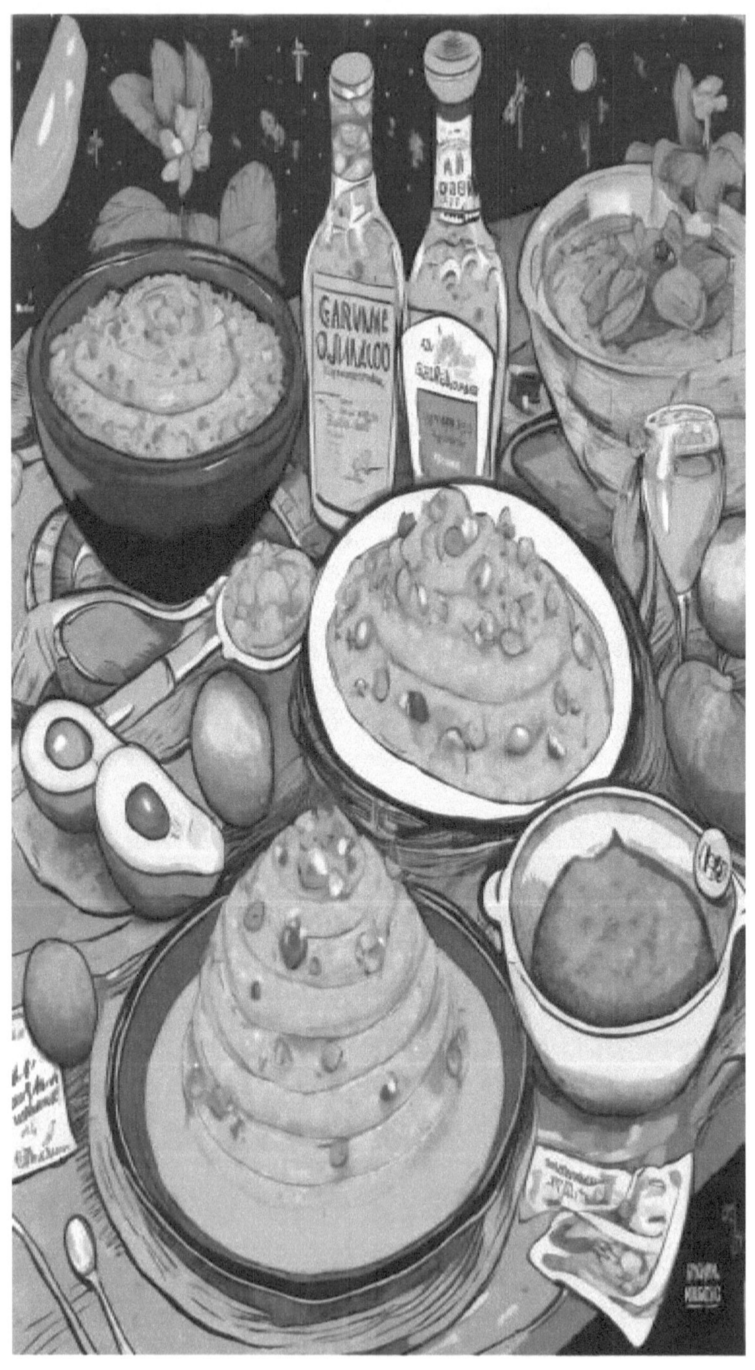

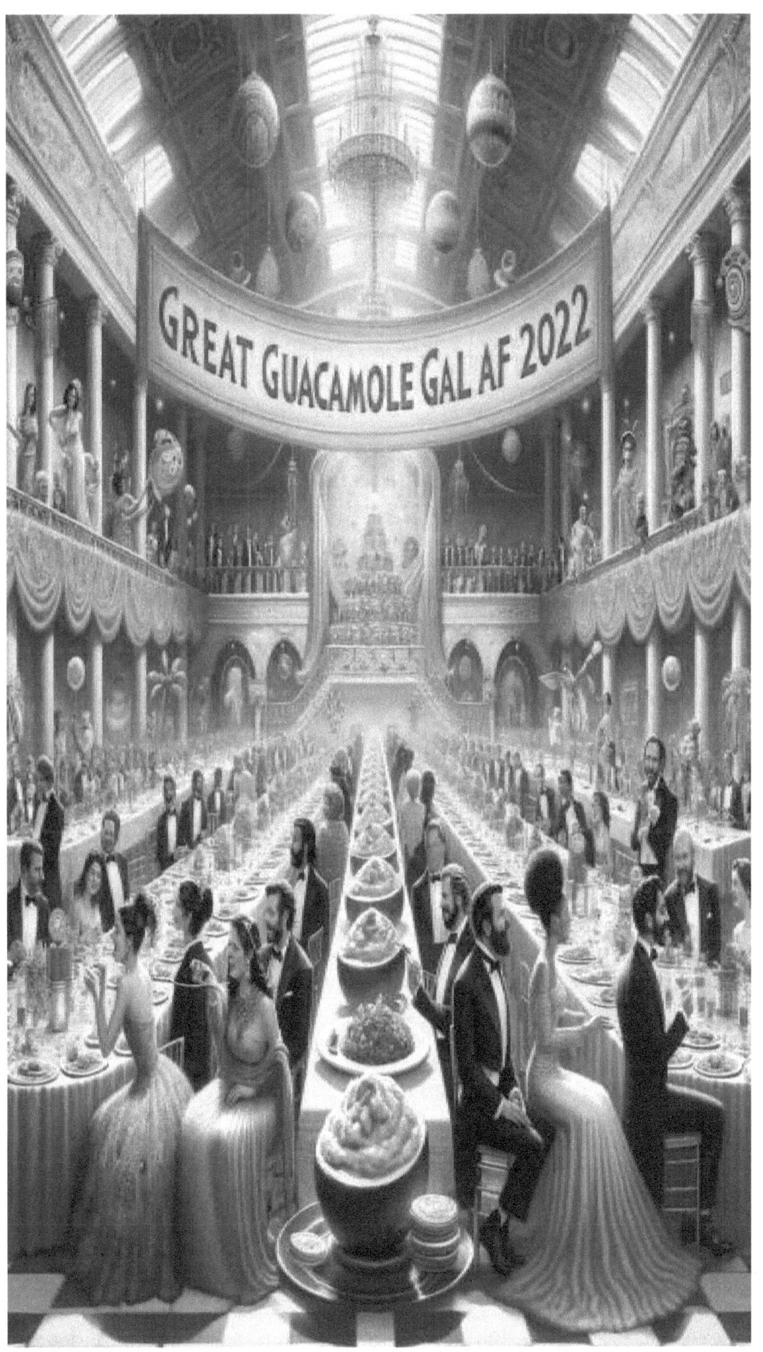

GREAT GUACAMOLE GAL AF 2022

The Great Guacamole Gala of 2023

In the tranquil, idyllic town of Avocadoville situated amidst sweeping landscapes, the annual, highly anticipated Guacamole Gala was the captivating event that notedly marked the year for all residents and visitors alike. Spearheaded by no lesser group than the internationally recognized organization, the Global Guacamole Group (GGG), this was the quintessential destination where individuals and enthusiasts, seeking to showcase their culinary excellence in creating guacamole, gathered in grandeur.

At the heart of Avocadoville's fervent community was our protagonist Granny Smith, a resident who held the revered title of Avocadoville's guacamole guru. Over an illustrious span of many years, Granny's unique and unparalleled recipe held a firm, glorious reign supreme, a favorite of all who tasted those green creamy scoops.

However, being a testament to the ever-evolving nature of life, this year introduced an unexpected, intriguing twist in the yearly gala. This twist came in the form of GGG's newest venture - venturing into the lip-puckering world of lime juice production. Their product? An exclusive brand dubbed "Lime Light." On the surface, it seemed innocent, but it came cloaked with a subtle condition. The GGG decided to contribute handsome donations to the gala but had a tiny string attached – only their new product, Lime Light, was permitted to be used in the esteemed competition.

Now, to understand this twist one must delve into the culinary world of guacamole. Every single aficionado, every guacamole connoisseur knows and emphasizes the colossal importance of lime in guacamole. It's the lively zing, the tangy zest, the electrifying pizzazz! But Granny Smith was a stalwart purist. She firmly believed in the traditional art of doing things. Her philosophy entitled the practice of squeezing her very own limes, maintaining that the manuals streak made all the noteworthy difference, adding a freshness that couldn't be rivaled.

When the much-anticipated gala day finally descended upon Avocadoville, poor Granny Smith's guacamole stand was largely overshadowed by blinding neon Lime Light ad banners and the distribution of free Lime Light shot glasses promoting the new product. The rest of the competitors, seduced by the generous support from GGG (and the undeniable allure of collecting those exquisite, free shot glasses) had succumbed to the pressure and meekly incorporated Lime Light into their age-old cherished recipes.

Tasting sessions added an extra layer of intrigue to the gala. Attendees sampled the various guacamoles presented, and to their surprise, an unexpected pattern emerged. The common critique being muttered was, "Tastes...overly limey?" However, the one glorious exception to this was at Granny Smith's inviting booth. Her alluring guacamole had retained its familiar, fresh zing and zest that everyone loved and craved, offering a stark contrast to the overpowering, flat lime onslaught resulting from the Lime Light inclusion.

When Granny Smith was awarded the trophy and crowned the competition's winner, murmurs of "sponsor bias" began to steadily arise amongst the crowd. While GGG's Lime Light indeed had its own merits (those free shot glasses standing testament to that), their undeniable influence over the gala's proceedings was crystal clear.

Reflections: This interesting event pushes us to acknowledge that much like in the nuanced, layered world of guacamole, when sponsors have an undeclared vested interest (or a new lime juice to sell, in this case), the core essence of an event or advocacy can subtly undergo an alteration. Whether the matters at action are ADHD advocacy groups or Guacamole galas, it becomes absolutely critical for the onlooker to discern genuine quality from what is simply a forceful squeeze from a vested interest.

As for our maverick Granny Smith, she remains inherently timeless and inimitable, now giving insightful workshops on the "Art of Lime Squeezing" – a strong testimony that proves that sometimes, sticking to the traditional way can retain its compelling zest even amidst rapidly urbanizing, modern pressures.

Chapter 6: Advocating for Big Pharma - The Influence of Industry Partnerships

Remember the tales your grandparents used to tell of bartering goods between villages? History repeats this timeless dance of partnerships in modern industry. Think back to the days when teams of innovative cavemen would collaborate to better their societies, trading one invention for something else of value; perhaps the wheel for a shiny, enticing rock that caught their eye. In today's global economic landscape, sophisticated versions of these age-old trading practices continue to shape our lives.

Speaking of shaping societal perspectives, patient advocacy organizations play an indispensable role. Just as members of a family listen to the wise old Aunt Agnes, who continuously takes the lead during family get-togethers, sharing her views on the most recent health concerns, similar to how these advocacy organizations influence public sentiment around critical health issues. Aunt Agnes has likely had her fair share of correct assumptions, although, every now and then, her judgment may be swayed by the allure of the free samples that door-to-door salesmen leave her. Reflecting on Attention Deficit Hyperactivity Disorder (ADHD), this presents a compelling parallel with established advocacy groups that have a history of creating partnerships with pharmaceutical stakeholders. While these collaborations have demonstrable benefits, they also come with their fair share of concerns around bias and impartiality that need addressing.

Let's take an interesting analogy to simplify this complex situation. Do you recall the sensational headline, "Ice Cream Causes Shark Attacks"? No? Allow me to jog your memory. As outlandish as it may sound initially, a peculiar statistical relationship was discovered between seemingly unrelated events - the increase in ice cream sales and the uptick in shark attacks. This absurdity, though, is quickly explained by a third variable: hot weather, leading to an increase in beach visits and thus a higher chance for shark attacks. This seemingly counter-intuitive example illustrates the principle of correlation versus causation. A similar example can be found in the healthcare sector involving ADHD advocacy groups. An article published in the esteemed journal Nature found that significant ADHD advocacy groups were recipients of substantial sponsorship from pharmaceutical companies with deep-seated commercial stakes (Rose, 2013). What does this suggest? Are these groups merely enjoying more chilled delicacies, or are they wading into shark-infested waters, metaphorically speaking? Financial support from these firms undoubtedly contributes to funding various initiatives; however, there is little to no transparency on the extent of the influence these financial contributions carry.

Let's try illustrating this concern with a bit of magical whimsy. Picture yourself in a room, captivated by the acts of a talented magician. With a sleight of hand, he pulls a rabbit out of an empty hat. You're impressed but left wondering, "Where did that rabbit come from?" This analogy resonates with a phenomenon in the world of nonprofit advocacy organizations where an obscure link seems to exist between monetary support from industry and the highlighting of the sponsors' products or services. In a comprehensive examination by the Journal of Medical Ethics, an issue termed "institutional corruption" is raised. This refers to a pattern where organizations, due to continuing dependance on financial sponsorship from corporations, end up veering away from their original missions and objectives, instead drifting towards the priorities of their backers (Cosgrove & Wheeler, 2013). It's much like our magician suddenly exclusively performing rabbit tricks, simply because the "International Rabbit Association" started to sponsor him.

Now let's move on to another interesting character from an imaginary chapter of my life: my twice-removed cousin, Benny. Benny, a master storyteller, had the remarkable knack of saying very little yet conveying extremely profound concepts. However, his vague narrative style always left you wondering about his real intentions or where he truly stood on issues. Regrettably, this enigma is not exclusive to fictional characters like Benny. It mirrors how many advocacy groups operate; their key priorities and motivations, too, often remain ambiguous. Lenzer (2018) provides an insightful observation that the recommendations of these organizations could potentially reflect the interests of their commercial partners more than those of the communities they claim to represent, due to limited disclosure of these relationships. You could argue these organizations embody Benny's elusive tendencies. Concerns often arise, doubting whether funded organizations manage to maintain their independence from their pharmaceutical benefactors or whether such relationships subtly shape the organizations' way of advocating.

Getting nostalgic about our childhood brings to mind sweet memories. Take my childhood friend, Timmy, for instance, known for his generous nature, regularly shared his candies. However, there was a catch to his generosity. Sometimes, he would pass you the black licorice, which was his least favorite, under the pretense of sharing. Similarly, patients deserve not simply the leftovers, but the advocacy which truly promotes their health and well-being, not guided merely by profit motives. It is crucial to ensure the beneficiaries of these advocacies aren't left confused, or worse, susceptible to potential harm when important information is veiled by commercial interests. For a balanced, effective advocacy, it is vital to establish a clear demarcation guaranteeing independence from commercial influence, through diversifying income sources, which would prevent any single entity from taking hold of the organization's objectives. In the same vein, you wouldn't want all your candy coming from one singular provider, especially when it's all licorice, would you? The cornerstone of accountability is transparency. When dealing with institutions that fulfill public roles, it is necessary to ensure transparency is not swept under the rug but held at the forefront where it most vitally needs to be.

Let's circle back to the story of Aunt Agnes. While her heart is certainly in the right place, she must remember her original purpose and resist being swayed by the allure of free samples. Advocacy organizations must safeguard the fundamental principle of integrity, accomplished through continuous vigilance and a willingness to adapt and reform as needed. The focus should be to wholeheartedly commit to providing objective guidance to their trusting constituents, devoid of any polarizing divide separating healthcare from commercial interests. The future of patient advocacy is contingent on nurturing the cooperation that truly fosters health. By avoiding opportunistic exploitation of vulnerabilities wherever they emerge, a meaningful, positive change can be brought about in public health. Let us not forget the lessons learnt from the licorice anecdote, always staying vigilant and questioning the motives behind what's being offered.

Time for Reflection:

1. **Objective vs. Influenced Advocacy**: Think about other advocacy organizations or movements you're familiar with.

How might their messaging be influenced if they were heavily funded by a vested interest? How would you differentiate between genuinely objective advice and potentially biased guidance?

2. **Transparency in Funding**: If you were to establish guidelines for transparency in funding for advocacy groups, what key elements would you include to ensure clarity and maintain trust among the general public?

3. **Balance of Power and Influence**: Reflect on the "institutional corruption" mentioned. How can advocacy organizations strike a balance between receiving necessary funding and maintaining their original mission? Are there examples from other sectors where organizations successfully navigated these waters?

4. **Personal Stake**: Consider a hypothetical situation where you or a loved one has ADHD. How would the relationship between pharmaceutical companies and advocacy groups influence your decisions or perceptions regarding treatment options? Would you feel confident in the advice provided by these groups knowing about potential industry ties?

References

Cosgrove, L., & Wheeler, E. E. (2013). Industry's colonization of psychiatry: Ethical and practical alternatives. The Catalyst, 33(1).

Lenzer, J. (2018). Financial ties between leaders of influential US professional medical associations and industry: cross-sectional study. BMJ, 361, k1516.

Rose, S. L. (2013). Patient advocacy organizations: Institutional conflicts of interest, trust, and trustworthiness. The Journal of Law, Medicine & Ethics, 41(3), 680-687.

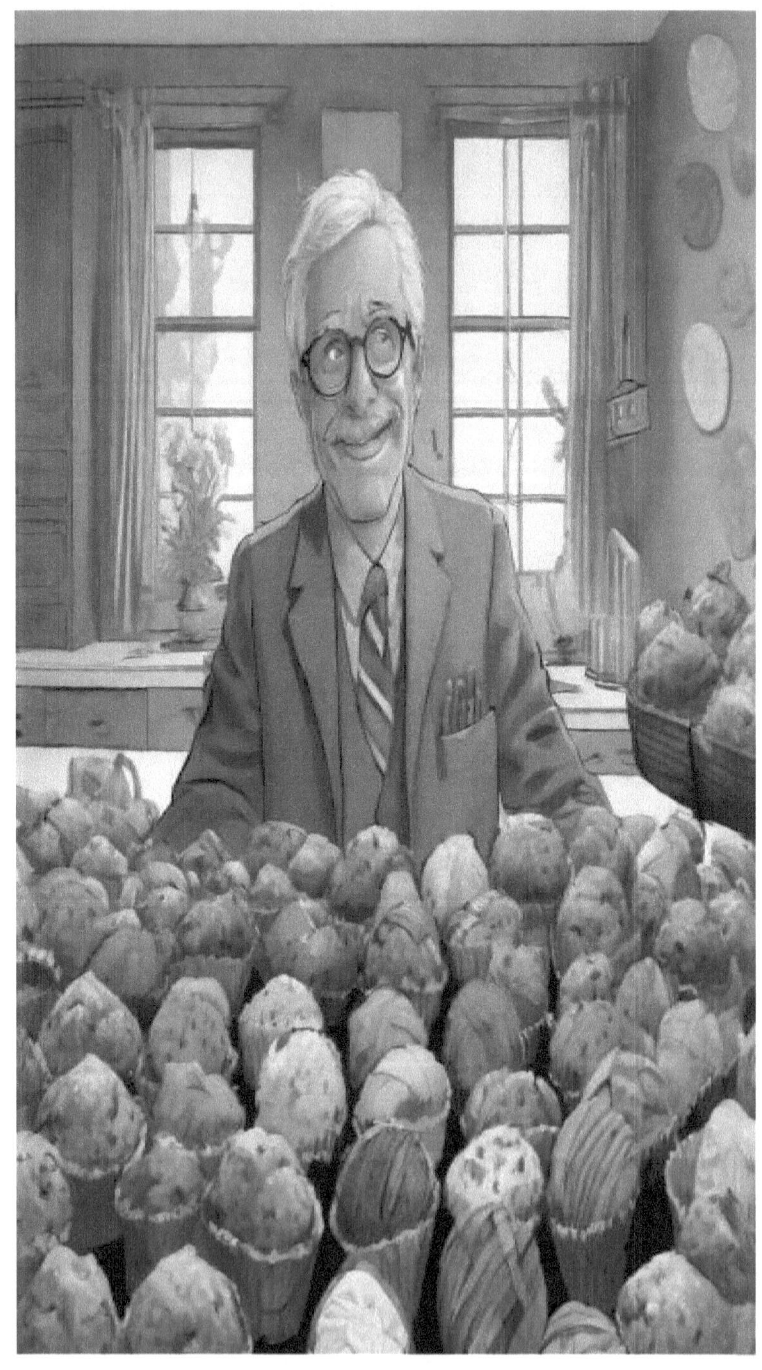

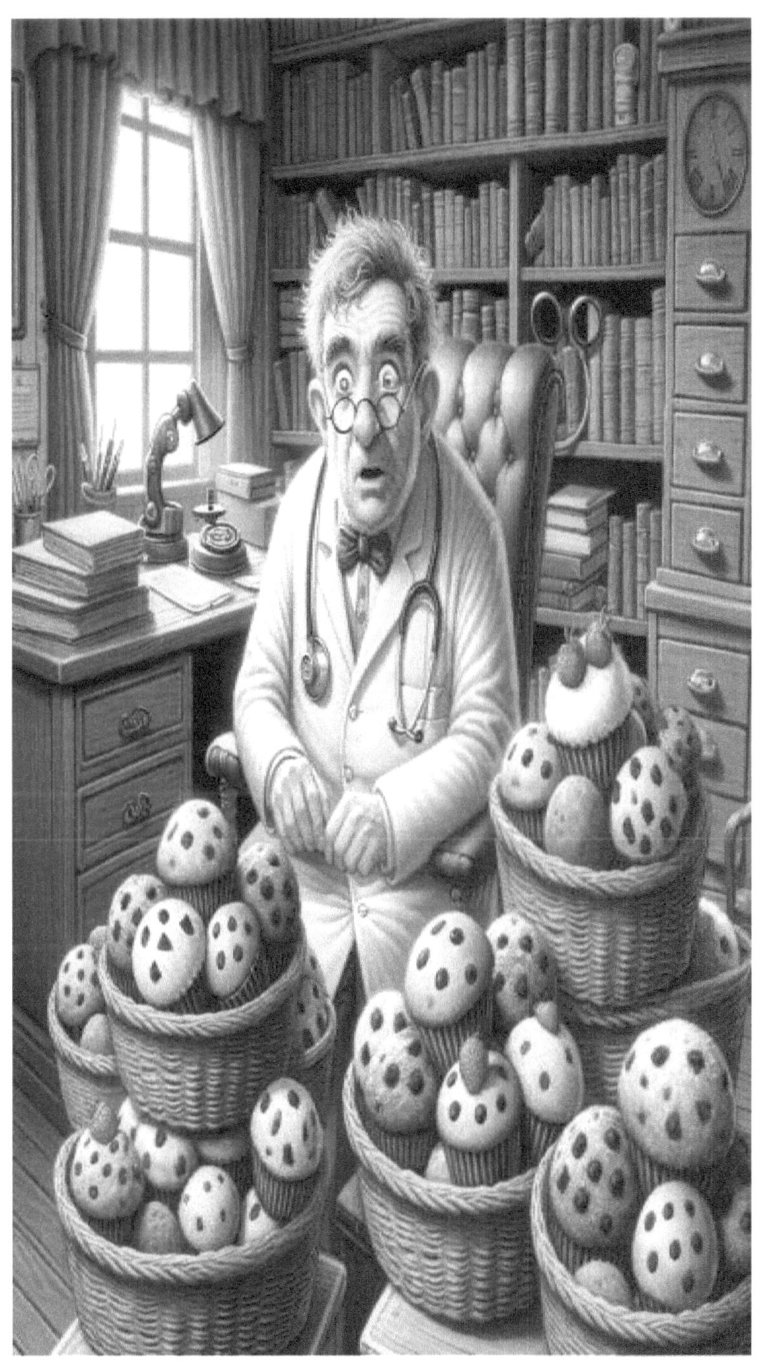

Dr. Monty and the Mysteriously Appearing Muffin Baskets

Introducing Dr. Monty Brownridge. He's not your typical physician. With years of experience under his belt, this seasoned and incredibly knowledgeable doctor has a unique personality - a refreshing blend of professionalism and friendly jollity. On top of being a competent physician, Dr. Monty is also a passionate gardener who finds immense joy in cultivating plants and an aficionado of lighthearted dad humor. Making his home in the quaint, close-knit community of Cloverville, he's been running a modestly sized medical practice that caters to the healthcare needs of the town's residents. He'd quickly become everyone's favorite healthcare provider due to his collection of brilliantly colored ties that mirrored his radiant spirit, and his amiable approach to treatment. From routine ailments to pressing existential dilemmas, Dr. Monty was a beacon of hope and support to all.

On one typical Monday morning, Dr. Monty was spotted tenderly watering 'Fernando,' his cherished office potted plant. Seated on his desk was an unexpected surprise - a basket teeming with delicious, homemade blueberry muffins. Tied to the basket was a gracious note from 'BestMed Pharma' - a pharmaceutical company - wishing him an enjoyable snack. Intrigued by the unexpected gift and never one to resist a good pastry, Monty eagerly bit into one of the muffins, sharing another with his dedicated assistant nurse, Patty. Following her lucky breakfast, Patty felt obligated to attend the seminar organized by 'BestMed Pharma' over the upcoming weekend.

During the seminar, Patty simultaneously managed to balance a plate heaped with more of those luscious muffins while attentively listening to a presentation detailing 'Revitoxin.' It was supposedly a revolutionary new medication, a miraculous remedy advertised to cure just about anything. In addition to the presentation, she was given attractive, glossy brochures that strangely enough, left out any mention of potential side effects. Energized by the seminar's proceedings, Patty returned to the clinic full of chatter about 'Revitoxin,' its presumed benefits, and of course, the irresistible blueberry muffins.

Dr. Monty, however, was a man who trusted only what came with clear instructions and a proven track record - just like his beloved plants. Skeptical about 'Revitoxin's' promising claims, he decided to investigate further. To his surprise, he uncovered that 'Revitoxin' had a dubious efficacy profile. Also, he found out that psychoeducation - a treatment approach that costed significantly less than the enticing muffins - was yielding more positive outcomes in treating many of the conditions 'Revitoxin' claimed to address.

Consequently, he waste no time in convening a meeting with his team. At this gathering, all muffin-based incentives were temporarily but emphatically vetoed. He expressed the importance of unbiased and holistic patient care. To preserve and foster medical integrity and objectivity, Monty formulated a strict "No Gifts" policy, which was meticulously followed. The only exceptions allowed were gifts of plant seeds, considering his fondness for gardening.

Moral of the story: The allure of a fluffy, heaven-sent muffin must not compromise the core of medical practice. Dr. Monty embodied the essential values of skepticism towards unknown sources and relentless adherence to prioritizing patient care, even in the face of tantalizing breakfast. He ensured the town of Cloverville learned a valuable lesson, 'Revitoxin' might not be the ultimate panacea it claimed to be, but one thing for sure, Dr. Monty's delightfully corny jokes could lighten any mood and might just be the best cure for the blues.

Chapter 7: Crafting the Message - Pharma's Influence on Healthcare Providers

The intricate and often convoluted dynamics we unwittingly find ourselves internalized within, the spiderweb-like entanglements that we expedite into existence - could this not also be applied, metaphorically, to the complex sphere of pharmaceutical representatives and their consistent stream of opulent and, sometimes, over-the-top lunch displays paraded before various doctors' offices? It seems a particularly surreal spectacle - one that, quite hilariously and yet disconcertingly, vibrates with all the alluring charm of a B-grade fantastical drama.

Back in the early epochs of my professional journey - in those so-called 'good old days' that pre-date the now obligatory proliferation of apps, and even precede the advent of patient reviews online - I vividly recall an instance of an unusually zealous drug rep. This representative, in an attempt to beguile our office with promises of a revolutionary new medicinal construct, decked out the meeting area with an assortment of themed cupcakes, followed by a painfully euphoric karaoke session that was, unfortunately, most decidedly off-key. And while this feels like a snippet straight out of comic folklore, we must always remember to view these actions in the appropriate light: these gestures are, more often than not, calculated and masterfully refined conduits towards serious and intricate goals.

The sphere of pharmaceutical lobbying is, by design, a particularly aggressive one, with these lobbyists attempting to strengthen their influence amongst the healthcare providers through various strategies. Such strategies include such mechanisms as continuing medical education seminars and detailing - which refers to the targeted visits made by drug representatives. Evidence collected through studies - particularly the one conducted by Fickweiler et al. in 2017 - have highlighted the troublesome correlation between direct financial links and non-objective prescribing. This situation is somewhat akin to having Aunt Martha persistently nudging you to invest in her friend's inchoate start-up, arguing passionately about the amazing deal she once received on a used car from said friend. While it would be delightful to assert our decisions are always grounded on the infallible pillars of data and necessity, we must confront the reality - that Aunt Martha's fruitcake often tastes unaccountably more delectable post her spirited pitch.

There's an inherent risk connected to such education-driven activities - that of emphasizing products peddled by the sponsors, rather than focusing on disseminating a balanced and comprehensive scientific inquiry as they merit. Imagine getting trapped into taking a free breakfast at a timeshare presentation, only to be overwhelmed by an incessant highlighting of why the particular timeshare – the one trying to sell you – is the optimum choice for you since the inception of sliced bread. Aptly reflecting the risk outlined here, speakers who have accepted funding from such sponsors do tend to preferentially zoom in on special interests - thereby shirking the unbiased medical advice that stakeholders heavily rely on.

It's indeed very similar to that vacation where, entranced by a beautifully styled brochure, you had made reservations, only to discover those breathtaking photos were perhaps a tad over-optimistic, shall we say? Transparently, this is the predicament that arises when one viewpoint is bestowed with an unbalanced portion of the spotlight. The narratives are more often focused on their branded drugs rather than discussing the comprehensive range of alternatives, such as psychoeducation - which, incidentally, has been proven to result in significant improvements in maintaining balance and enhancing resiliency.

Physicians possess a considerable amount of power and influence. However, for patient trust to be unswerving, they must demonstrate their independence from commercial interests. To build on this argument, I offer the example of trusting your barber: you wouldn't want them giving you a mullet hairstyle simply because a particular hair product company provides them a better deal on products that favor the mullet look, would you? It's transparent, therefore, how relationships should exist free of vested commercial considerations that may undermine crucial objectivity.

Physicians should critically analyze and consider all perspectives through a diligent review process that's free from bias by promotional interests. A simple analogy helps illustrate this concept: consider for a moment a world where you were limited to only check out a film review written by its producer's mother. It is clear, then, that individualized care should take into account a robust range of options rather seeing the focus limited to the single area of product emphasis. When it comes to safeguarding clinical freedom against undue external pressures, whether these pressures be of a legislative or self-regulatory nature, appropriate policy forms the bulwark that protects the sacrosanct responsibilities that form the very core of the medical profession itself.

To conclude, the idea of accepting a complimentary pen or a free sandwich may seem inconsequential. Nevertheless, the implications of accepting these supposedly minor offerings can indeed hold profound implications on our practice. As the gatekeepers of healthcare, it's our bounden duty to safeguard the health of patients, unequivocally positioning it as the topmost priority, always. The side-splitting karaoke presentations? Perhaps they should be limited strictly to the weekends, don't you think?

Time for Reflection:

1. **Influence & Objectivity:** Think of a time when you were offered something "for free" or a favor in return for a seemingly simple action. How did it influence your decision-making, even subconsciously? Can you draw parallels to how physicians might feel when approached by pharmaceutical reps?

2. **Balanced Inquiry:** Consider the sources of health or medical information you've relied upon in the past. Were they impartial? How can you ensure a balanced perspective in future medical decisions, knowing that even professionals may be subjected to industry biases?

3. **Trust & Independence:** How do you personally evaluate the trustworthiness and independence of a medical professional or a health source? Has this chapter influenced how you might assess this trustworthiness in the future?

4. **Policy & Practice:** Reflect on the policies and guidelines that your healthcare provider, or a healthcare provider you know, has in place. Are they adequate to protect both the provider's and patients' interests from undue external influences? If not, what changes would you recommend?

References

Fickweiler, F., Fickweiler, W., & Urbach, E. (2017). Interactions between physicians and the pharmaceutical industry generally and sales representatives specifically and their association with physicians' attitudes and prescribing habits: a systematic review. PLOS Medicine, 14(9), e1002361.

Pliszka, S. R. (2007). Practice parameter for the assessment and treatment of children and adolescents with attention-deficit/hyperactivity disorder. Journal of the American Academy of Child & Adolescent Psychiatry, 46(7), 894-921.

Sah, S., & Fugh-Berman, A. (2013). Physicians under the influence: Social psychology and industry marketing strategies. The Journal of Law, Medicine & Ethics, 41(3), 665-672.

Sismondo, S. (2007). Ghost management: How much of the medical literature is shaped behind the scenes by the pharmaceutical industry? PLOS Medicine, 4(9), e286.

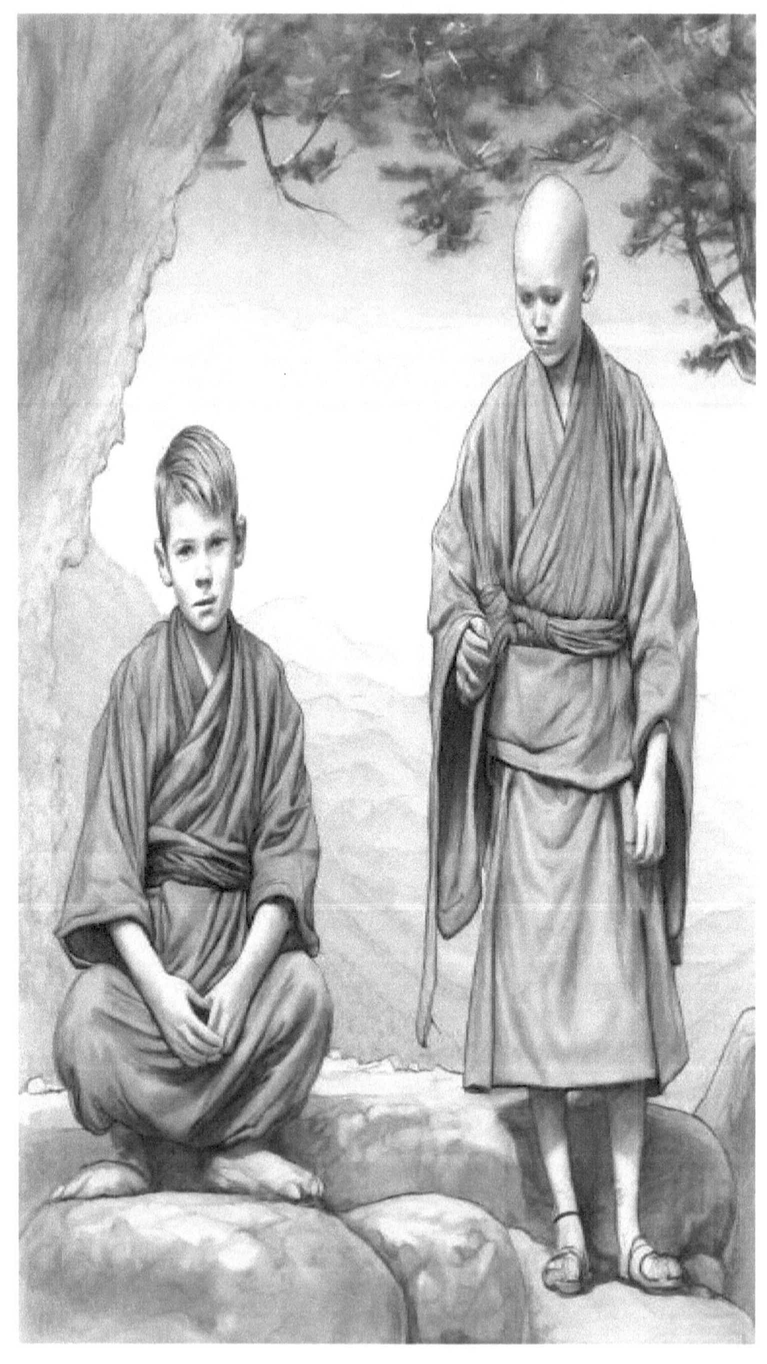

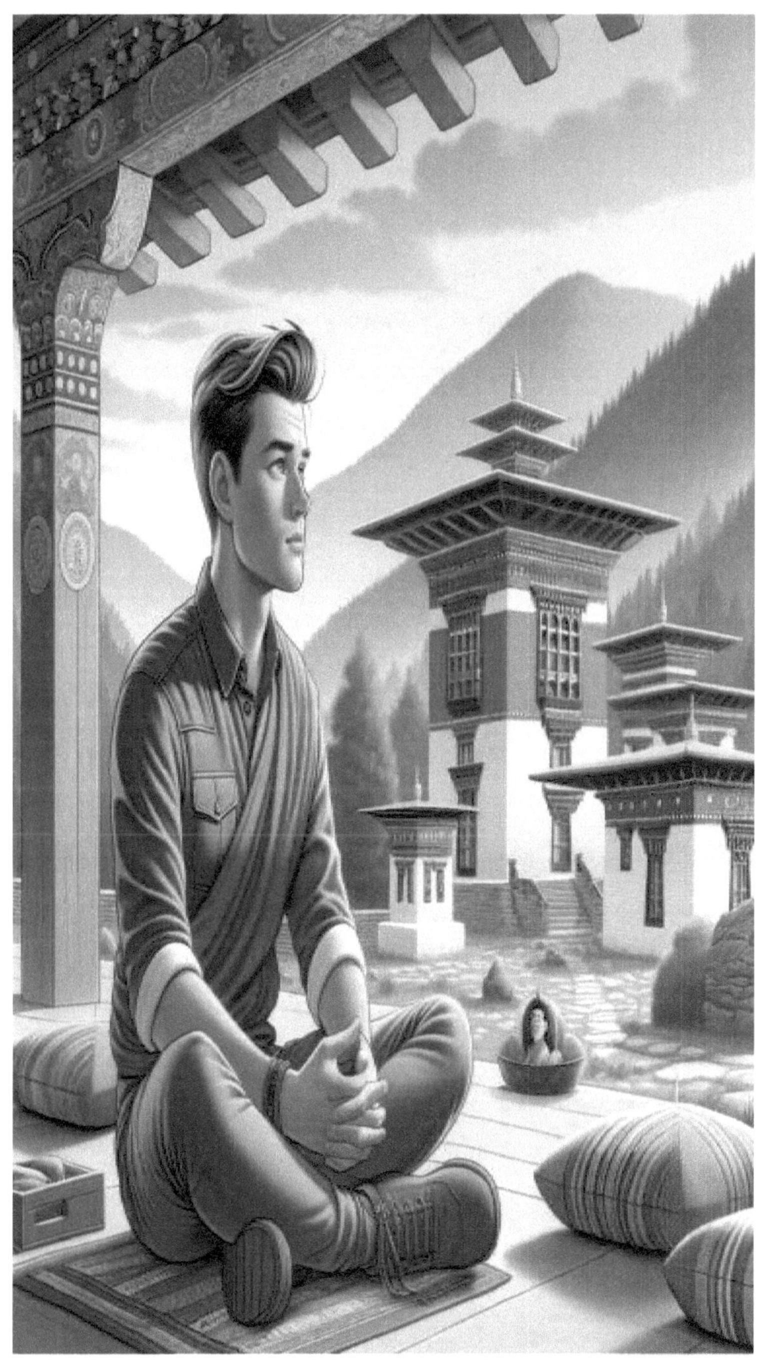

The Curious Case of Bubbly Billy in Bhutan

Immersed deep within the serene haven of the Himalayan enclave of Bhutan, where the measure of Gross National Happiness revered far above Gross Domestic Product, there existed an effervescent character named Bubbly Billy. Born in the bustling metropolis of Boston, Billy found himself transplanted to the quiet serenity of Bhutan as a young child, accompanying his parents who were passionate researchers. Billy was renowned for his unparalleled dynamism and ceaseless energy. During his time in Boston, his educators would often suggest that he might be grappling with an ADHD diagnosis. However, in Bhutan, his boundless vigor was met with smiles and a comparison to a lively, energetic yak in the blossoming period of Spring.

One luminous day, a representation of the Western pharmaceutical industry ventured into the tranquil valleys of Bhutan. This was a pharmaceutical representative, christened Pharma Phil, who introduced himself into the community equipped with glossy brochures and samples of ADHD medication, his tools of trade. His purpose was to hold a workshop, dramatically and metaphorically titled, "Taming the Wild Yaks: Understanding ADHD." This intriguing title indeed captured the attention of many Bhutanese, igniting curiosity yet aggression in equal measure. Others decided to remain skeptical and wondered if Pharma Phil might have just been overindulging himself with copious amounts of the local butter tea.

In the midst of his workshop, an alert Bhutanese teacher boldly rose, voiced a comment that left the room in an uproar of laughter. The teacher's simple suggestion was a reflection of the Bhutanese perspective, "You refer to it as ADHD; we consider it potential monk material!" Despite the thunderous laughter that ripped through the room, Pharma Phil maintained his professional etiquette. He continued his presentation unperturbed, emphasizing with the focused gravitas, the urgent need to diagnose and provide the necessary treatment for the condition.

In the aftermath of Pharma Phil's contentious presentation, Billy's parents found themselves at a crossroads of sorts. In Boston, there was the clinical option of medication to manage Billy's energy, yet in Bhutan, they were surrounded by a society that embraced patience as its virtue. After considering their options at great lengths, the parents decided to seek advice from a wise local monk. His profound yet simple counsel was, "Permit Billy to simply be Billy. Just as the magnificent landscapes around us, the mountains weren't shaped in just a single day."

Bubbly Billy's journey quickly transformed into a well-known legend etched into the narrative of Bhutan, emerging as a vibrant symbol of the clash between the aggressive Western pharmaceutical industry and the quaint local wisdom prevalent in Bhutan. Having witnessed this stark cultural contrast, Pharma Phil left Bhutan with a new level of wisdom and understanding, and an unexpected fondness for the local butter tea. As for Billy? He found his calling as a tour guide, harnessing his ceaseless energy into showcasing the stunning beauty of Bhutan to eager visitors. He ensured that everyone who set foot in this land left with their happiness quotient a little higher than when they arrived.

Chapter 8: Expanding Markets - Big Pharma's Global Influence

The invaluable advantages that a broader understanding can offer are available to all of us; however, it is often the case that the focal points of the pharmaceutical industry can have significant implications on cross-cultural diagnoses. In an effort to better illustrate this concept, allow me to transport you back in time to one of my most memorable experiences during a global symposium.

Among the attendees was an affable senior gentleman from none other than the city of love itself, France. In the interest of preserving this individual's privacy, let's refer to him as Pierre. Sporting a friendly smile, Pierre approached me with a bottle of vintage French wine in one hand and a scholarly paper, concentrated on detailing ADHD, on the other. Recalling his distinctive French accent, he said, "You see, in our beautiful France, we used to look upon ADHD as mere signs of lively children; but now, voilà! We seem to be immediately reaching for medications at any hint of ADHD!" His words underscored how psycho-pharmaceutical cooperation disseminates Western concepts of mental health disorders globally, broadening access but simultaneously amplifying requests for medications (Storebø et al., 2018).

Ah, the wonders of globalization! It crafts an image of a world where a teenager situated in the bustling city of Tokyo could very well be relishing a Big Mac – a decidedly Western delicacy – while adopting Western drugs at the very hint of ADHD symptoms. However, it's worth noting that globalization isn't merely about amalgamating diverse perspectives into a global marketplace, but rather, it typically prioritizes profit over the crucial subtleties of cultural variances.

My esteemed colleague Dr. Ramon often humorously opined that if one were to take a global map and plot the expansion of ADHD diagnoses, it wouldn't be unlike tracing the well-trodden paths of hardworking pharmaceutical sales representatives. Recent research studies have hinted at a significant connection between the rise in international ADHD diagnoses and the intensifying collaboration between pharmaceutical corporations (Elbe & Caraça, 2020). Dr. Ramon would then assert, half in jest, "Looks like they might actually be more effective at their jobs than us medical professionals!" However, jokes aside, these observations underscore the mounting necessity of establishing efficient oversight measures, not only globally, but also within our domestic healthcare systems.

While cultural perceptions towards health and illness often display distinct differences, it's no secret that the universal drive for profits tends to impose a pressure towards uniformity. This brings to mind an intriguing anecdote from a trip I took to Japan for a medical conference. During a casual evening outing, a local psychiatrist, after a round of sake, revealed, "Truthfully, we Japanese never really endorsed the concept of ADHD. But now, it's become a condition everyone seems to desire a diagnosis for – quite like a popular sushi roll!" Irrespective of Japan's initial skepticism towards ADHD, despite the relentless marketing efforts of various pharmaceutical corporations, diagnoses of the condition have seen a sudden upsurge (Schor, 2011). And it is strikingly apparent that this unprecedented popularity of ADHD diagnoses mirrors financial motivations rather than the genuine needs of the country's population. Historical medical frameworks and treatment methodologies run the risk of fading away when driven by profit-oriented globalization. This is somewhat reminiscent of how my grandmother's cherished secret cookie recipe almost faced oblivion when a large-scale bakery attempted to commercialize it – a situation that may not equate perfectly to healthcare globalization, but it certainly illuminates the overarching principle.

One of the key requirements of ethical global health care is the acknowledgement and respect towards indigenous knowledge and practices. During one of my travels, I happened to meet a wise shaman from Bhutan who said, "While you choose to manage ADHD with medications, we, on the other hand, prefer to address it with understanding and patience." This profound perspective prompts some sober reflection. Commercial interests and clinical priorities, as it turns out, do not always walk hand in hand. They tend to diverge particularly when the driving force is financial gain rather than genuine medical necessity.

Initiatives aimed at enhancing access to medication should ideally be executed like a beautifully choreographed dance – masterfully balancing universal access privileges with an individualized understanding that is entirely dependent on location-specific cultures and traditions. A healthy international collaboration functions similarly – much like a great potluck. It thrives not only by selling, but also by mutually sharing enriching experiences and knowledge, in turn combining potential financial gains with the richness of societal benefits. This also serves as a poignant reminder of Pierre's words, often accompanied by his signature blend of wine and ADHD research: "Balance, my friend, is indeed the essence of life."

Time for Reflection:

1. **Pharmaceutical Priorities vs Cultural Perspectives**: Considering the spread of Western medical constructs, in what ways might pharmaceutical priorities overshadow or interact with a culture's traditional understanding of behavioral and psychological conditions?

2. **Economic Influence on Diagnosis**: How do you perceive the relationship between financial interests of pharmaceutical companies and the rise in ADHD diagnoses in countries previously skeptical of the condition? Can you think of other instances in healthcare where economic interests might influence medical decisions?

3. **Local Expertise and Global Health**: Reflecting on the anecdote about the shaman in Peru, how do local healing practices and beliefs provide valuable perspectives, and how can these be integrated or respected alongside modern medical practices?

4. **Balancing Universal Rights with Individualized Understanding**: How can global health initiatives promote a harmonious balance between providing access to treatments while also respecting cultural individualities and local expertise? What challenges might arise, and how can they be addressed?

References

Elbe, S., & Caraça, J. (2020). Rethinking global health governance in an era of multiple crises. Global Policy, 11(1), 1-9.

Schor, E. L. (2011). Policymaking in schools of medicine as viewed through the lens of pharmaceutical marketing. Academic Medicine, 86(2), 129-134.

Storebø, O. J., Ramstad, E., Krogh, H. B., Nilausen, T. D., Skoog, M., Holmskov, M., ... & Moreira-Maia, C. R. (2018). Methylphenidate for children and adolescents with attention deficit hyperactivity disorder (ADHD). Cochrane Database of Systematic Reviews, (2).

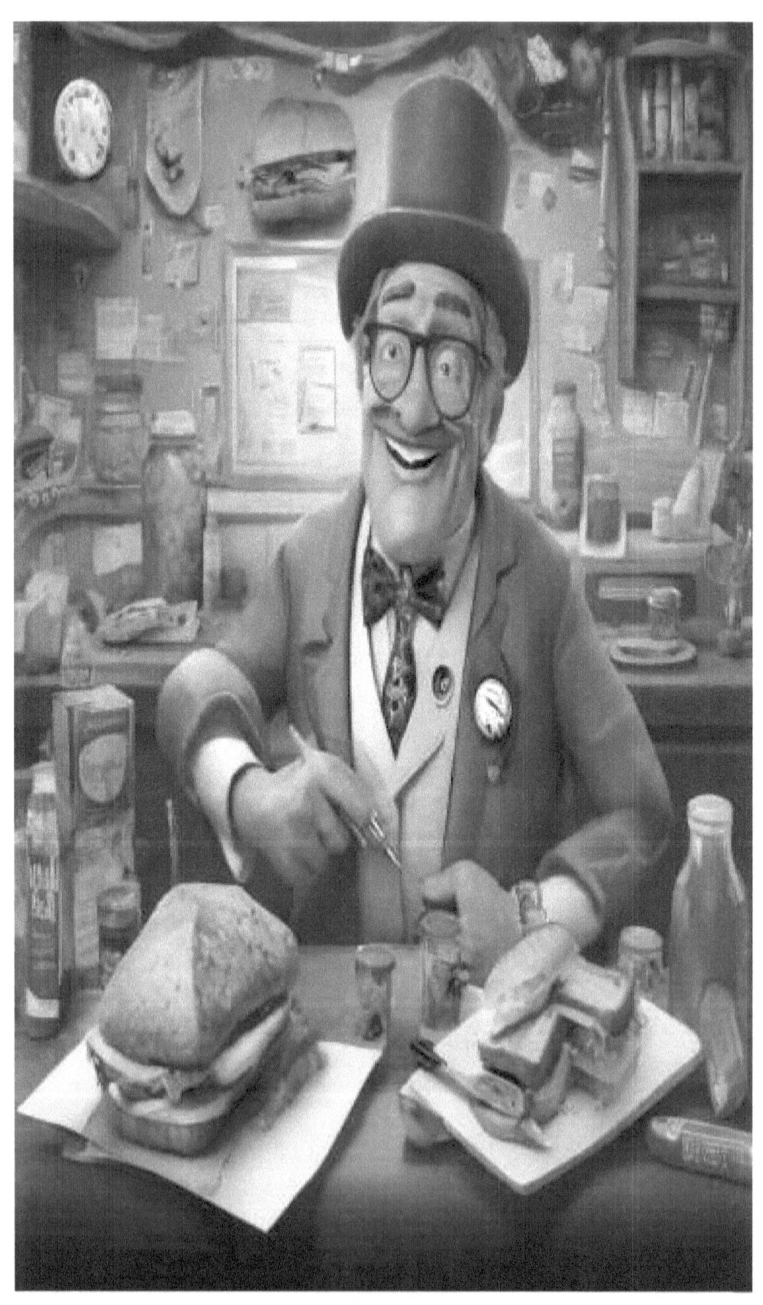

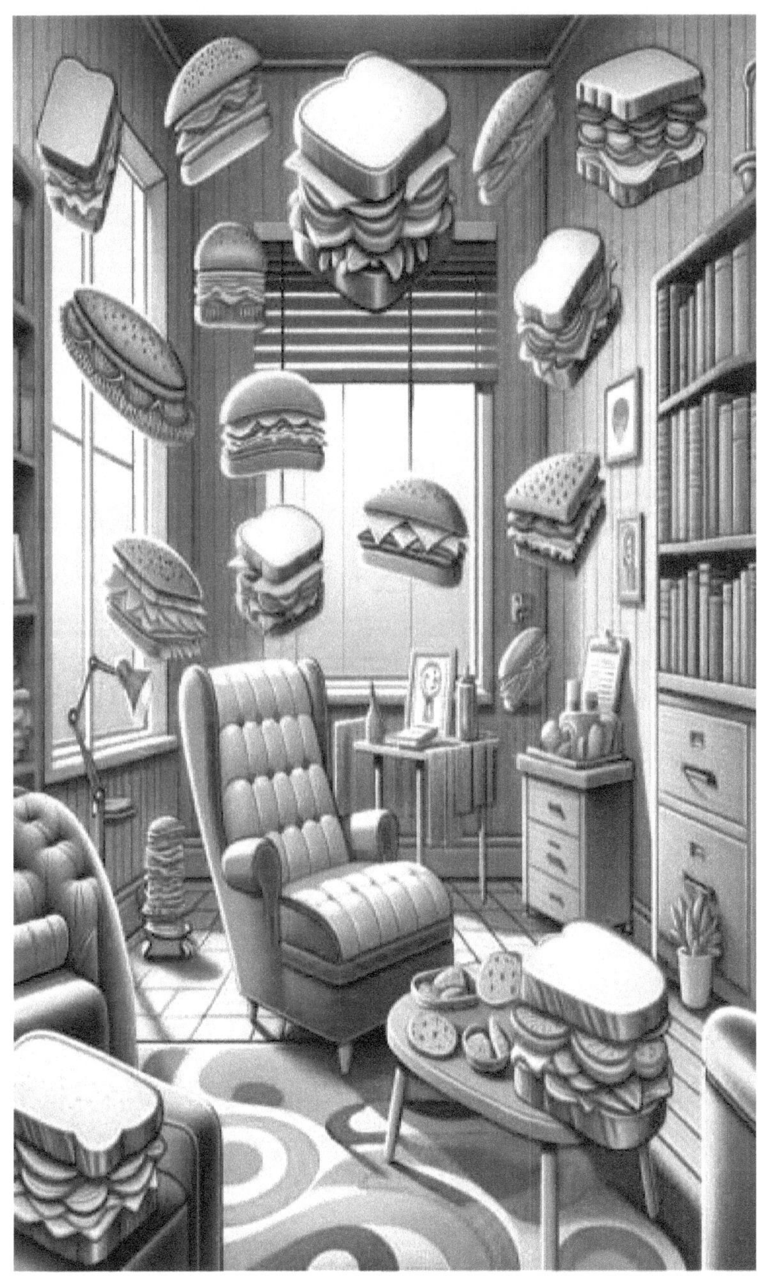

Dr. Phil McCrackin's Wild Ride with "PillPal" Promos

Setting the scene: Our tale unfurls in the cozy, small and delightful town of Medville. A community with its own unique charm, the place is famed and celebrated for its yearly custom - the syringe festival. A seemingly strange tradition to outsiders, but to its cheerful inhabitants, it's the highlight of their social calendar. However, Medville is also notorious in the annals of history for an infamous incident in 1998, fondly remembered as the "Cough Drop Caper". Indeed, the memory of this event still elicits a shiver down the spine of even the oldest town occupants.

Our protagonist: Step forward, Dr. Phil McCrackin. This charismatic and well-beloved psychiatrist is a distinct figure in the town, both for his professional prowess and his peculiar personal traits. Sporting a quirky attraction toward anything glaringly shiny, Dr. McCrackin has a weakness that many people find somewhat endearing – he has an irresistible penchant for gourmet sandwiches.

Situation: Into this peaceful scenery, the name "PillPal Pharmaceuticals" comes to hold significance. Not hesitating to capitalize on Dr. McCrackin's known attributes, the pharmaceutical company advanced with a lucrative proposal as irresistible as a savory cheesecake beautifully displayed at a diet convention. The offer included enticing speaking fees, an unlimited sandwich card (a surefire swoon for McCrackin given his weakness for delicious sandwiches), and an ornate pen which had the dual function of doubling as a disco light. The offer was greeted with warmth and accepted in kind.

An unexpected development: Anonymously, about a month into this cozy "partnership," our dear Doctor begins noticing some perplexing patterns. The scenario that repeats itself time and again is this – each time he writes a prescription for "FocusFast" (an ADHD remedy which is the latest brainchild of PillPal), he finds himself instinctively reaching for his new, flashy pen. A pure happenstance? So believed Dr. McCrackin initially. Until the day arrived when he caught himself absent-mindedly chanting, "PillPal's the best, forget the rest," in the middle of writing a prescription.

The Intervention of Regulatory Reinforcements:

1. *Disclosure Requirements*: Influenced by these incidents, Dr. McCrackin was thrust into a position where he was required to prominently display a badge bearing the inscription, "Proudly Sponsored by Sandwiches & PillPal." This instigated a new

dilemma. His patients started questioning the motivation behind the "FocusFast" prescriptions. Was it for their medical benefit or was it simply a means for the Doctor to satiate his love for sandwiches?

2. *Clinical Practice Guidelines*: The Medville Medical Association, keen to ensure transparency and integrity, enforced new laws requiring all staff to make public conflict-of-interest declarations. The well-loved Dr. McCrackin now found himself confessing his unwavering love for sandwiches at every seminar where he advocated for ADHD treatments. The result was a mixture of mirth and justified concern. Many found humor in his confession, but they made doubly sure to scrutinize all "FocusFast" prescriptions.

3. *Limits on Gifts*: Regulatory changes spelled a new chapter - PillPal couldn't provide gourmet sandwiches anymore. Their offerings were now limited to plain bread with a modest smear of butter. Disappointed and sandwich-deprived, Dr. McCrackin saw his once prized flashy disco pen collect dust, its charm having worn out.

4. *Prescription Data Privacy Laws*: PillPal found itself deprived of access to Dr. McCrackin's prescribing behavior. This resulted in a stop to the "special discounts" on "FocusFast," which were previously offered to McCrackin based on the frequency and quantity of prescriptions he made. The company had to grapple with the fact that no strings attached could also translate into less gain.

5. *Post-approval Drug Studies*: An unexpected revelation made things even more complicated - "FocusFast," praised for its ability to enhance focus, had a rather strange side-effect. A whopping 80% of its users developed an unusual craving for, yes, sandwiches! The irony of this discovery caused many to raise their eyebrows and chuckle.

Conclusion: Although the entire saga involving Dr. McCrackin and his relationship with sandwiches could be painted with a humorous brush, it served an important function; casting light on the influence of Big Pharma and the need for regulations. It was not too long after these events that such laws and regulations were affectionately christened "McCrackin's Laws" in Medville. They served as a tangible reminder to both medical professionals and patients that, despite the temptation of juicy sandwiches, paramount value and priority should be always placed on patient care. After all, the well-being and health of patients should never be compromised or sandwiched between the personal gains of a doctor and pressures from pharmaceutical companies.

Chapter 9 - Limiting Big Pharma's Influence through Regulation

Regulation. Maybe it's not a topic that would set the room alight in a social setting. It would probably score alongside watching paint dry in terms of excitement. Yet, just as the paint serves as the crucial protective and decorative layer for a wall, regulation in our socio-economic environment serves as an essential safeguard, a mechanism that keeps many elements of society operating within acceptable norms. Now imagine stripping a wall of its paint; you have an exposed wall, open to the mercy of the elements. Similarly, a world without regulatory norms would be as awkward and vulnerable as a freshman on their very first day in a public speaking class.

The role that Big Pharma plays in society - a role that stretches far beyond the boundaries of mere healthcare - has lately been the subject of a fair bit of critical examination. Policymakers are increasingly feeling the heat, a mounting pressure to step in and rein in what are viewed by many as excessive, overreaching actions by the pharmaceutical industry. To put this into the simplest, most basic terms, imagine you're back in school. Think of that one over-zealous kid on the playground who always tried to thrust candy bars in your face, trying to get you to buy one. Now, think of the school authorities stepping in to prevent this sort of thing, to ensure that the other kids don't end up eating candy bars for breakfast, lunch, and dinner.

To manage the deep, far-reaching reach of Big Pharma and to optimally utilize the immense resources that the pharmaceutical industry has at its disposal, while at the same time ensuring that the welfare of patients remains a constant priority, a number of strategies may be employed:

Firstly, there's the strategy of imposition of disclosure requirements. These are essentially regulations that necessitate physicians to come clean about financial ties that they may have with the industry – like they would have to declare the fact that they received speaker fees from a pharmaceutical company. This is perfectly comparable to a teacher disclosing a potential conflict of interest – say, for instance, a teacher who is also the parent of a student in the class. Here's a ready example: A friend of mine, Dr. Bob, who once accepted a pen as a gift from a pharmaceutical rep. Now, whenever Dr. Bob would use that pen to write a prescription, he'd laugh a bit, saying something like, "I feel so sponsored right now!" Although this type of transparency isn't perfect, it does build awareness and gives some insight into existing biases (Lundh et al., 2017).

Next we have clinical practice guidelines. These are a useful set of regulations that impose a duty on physicians to make clear conflict-of-interest statements. Consider this analogy: Aunt Millie, famed for her wonderful brownies, once made a batch for the school bake sale. However, she neglected to mention one tiny detail - these were actually "special" brownies. Little bits of information can be enormously helpful, as Aunt Millie's infamous bake sale demonstrated. The idea here is essentially to establish an informed consensus regarding the best patient care strategies over and above the commercial considerations (American Psychiatric Association, 2013).

Then there are the limitations imposed on the goodies, often employed as a tactic to sway judgement. This covers gifts, free meals, and promotional swag. Imagine this: a representative from a pharmaceutical company presents you with an exuberantly expensive meal, and before you know it, you're hooked and are prescribing their specific products left, right, and center like you're Oprah shouting, "You get a drug! And you get a drug!" Curbing such soft coercion tactics is crucial to maintaining clinical objectivity, to keep our inner Oprah under control, and above all, to put patient welfare firmly in the foreground (Dana & Loewenstein, 2003; Kesselheim et al., 2010).

Prescription data privacy laws are another important set of regulations in our arsenal. These can be thought of as the bouncers of the Big Pharma club, effectively keeping out intruders from mining in-house prescription data to better tailor their promotional strategies. No one likes the uncomfortable feeling of being profiled, and this is truer in the medical field than anywhere else. Protecting privacy means ensuring that our private medical data is as securely locked up as a teenager's diary, keeping unwelcome hands away and offering protection from any unwarranted shaping of medical interactions (O'Connor, 2019).

Finally, the pharmaceutical equivalent of the school progress report: post-approval drug studies and data registries. Think of it as a teacher asking for a follow-up on a student long after an assignment has been turned in. It's important to know if a patient such as Johnny, started experiencing unusual side effects after taking a new ADHD medication, like sprouting a third arm (heaven forbid!). This is critical for spotting long-term risks that might otherwise be downplayed by companies, such as metabolic changes from extended stimulant use (Castellanos & Proal, 2012; Shaw et al., 2009).

In sum, none of these strategies is a silver bullet, a one-size-fits-all solution. We don't live in a Willy Wonka world, after all. However, with a consistent revision of policies through open dialogues grounded in evidence, we can find a middle ground balancing the needs and wants of the pharmaceutical industry and the broader public health objectives. Just possibly, we can prevent Big Pharma from defining who supposedly has ADHD and who doesn't. Let's all lift a glass to that ideal!

Time for Reflection:

1. **On Transparency:** Have you ever been influenced by someone's undisclosed motives, be it in the medical field or elsewhere? How would knowing their affiliations or potential biases ahead of time have changed your perspective or decisions?

2. **Guidelines & Conflict of Interest:** When thinking about the balance between commercial priorities and optimal care, can you recall a situation where this balance was skewed? How do you believe conflict-of-interest statements could have impacted this situation?

3. **Gifts & Influences:** Reflect on a time you might have been swayed by a gift or gesture. In the realm of healthcare, why do you think it's especially crucial for professionals to remain uninfluenced by such offerings?

4. **Data Privacy & Long-Term Impacts:** How would you feel if your personal prescription data was used to target you with specific drugs or treatments? Similarly, do you think

the healthcare industry does enough to monitor the long-term effects of medications after they've been approved? What more could be done?

References

American Psychiatric Association. (2013). DSM-5 Task Force Disclosure. Washington, DC: Author.

Castellanos, F. X., & Proal, E. (2012). Large-scale brain systems in ADHD: beyond the prefrontal–striatal model. Trends in cognitive sciences, 16(1), 17-26.

Dana, J., & Loewenstein, G. (2003). A social science perspective on gifts to physicians from industry. JAMA, 290(2), 252-255.

Kesselheim, A. S., Robertson, C. T., Myers, J. A., Rose, S. L., Gillet, V., Roumiantseva, P., ... & Avorn, J. (2013). The costs of self-referral in health insurance: Evidence from legislative attempts to curb physician self-referral in the US. Health Policy Review, 3(3), 324-345.

Lundh, A., Lexchin, J., Mintzes, B., Schroll, J. B., & Bero, L. (2017). Industry sponsorship and research outcome. Cochrane Database of Systematic Reviews, 2.

O'Connor, C. (2019, January 16). Privacy advocates warn HHS not to share Americans' health records with researchers. Stat. https://www.statnews.com/2019/01/16/hhs-health-records-data-privacy/

Shaw, P., et al. (2009). Long-term effects of methylphenidate on cortical thickness in children with attention deficit hyperactivity disorder. Biological Psychiatry, 66(3), 216-223.

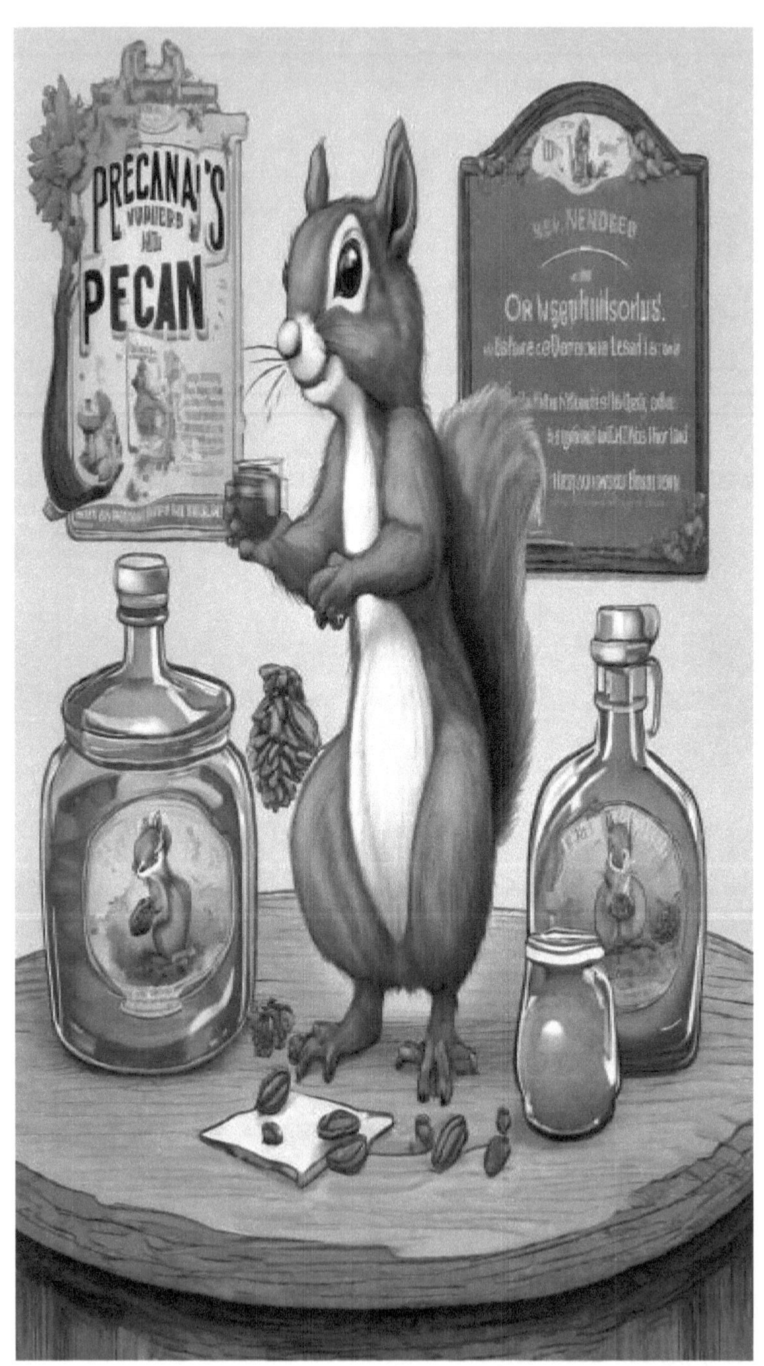
PRECANAL'S
PECAN

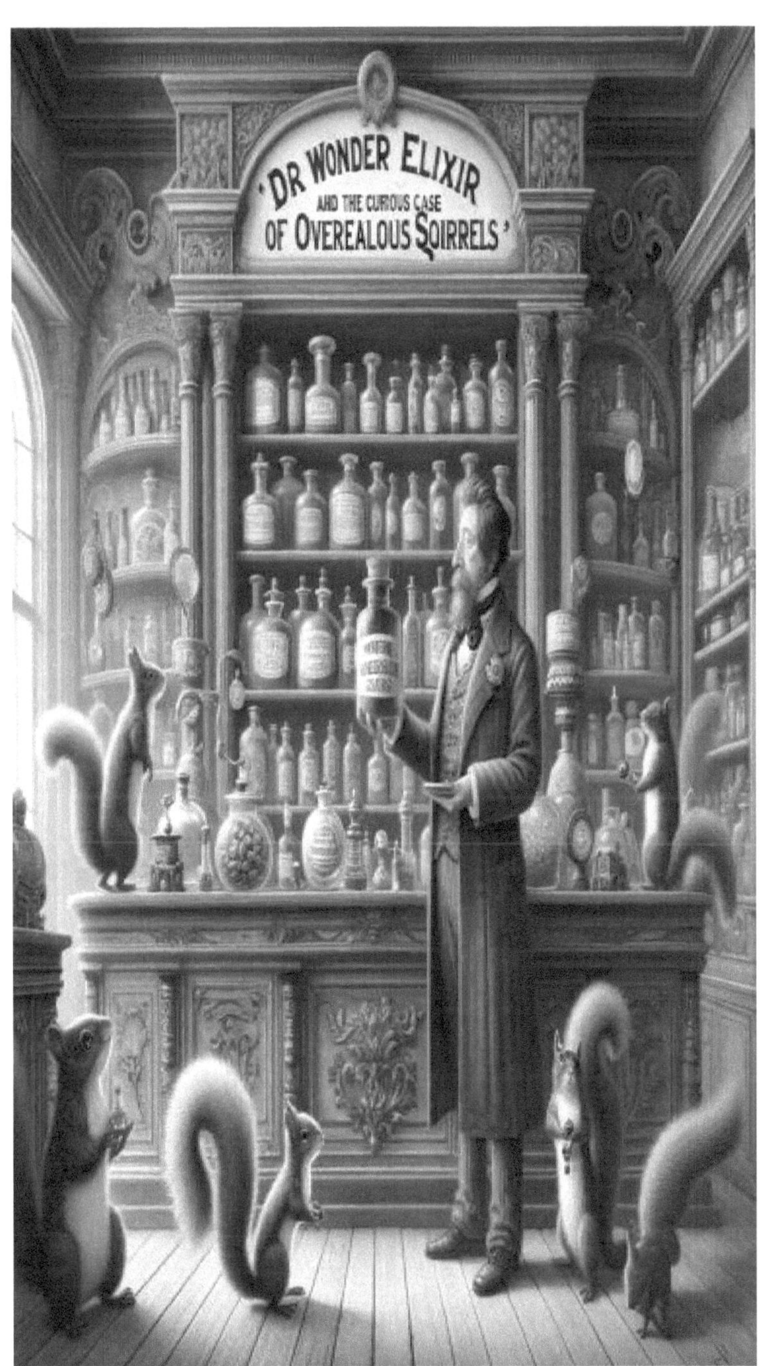

'DR WONDER ELIXIR
AND THE CURIOUS CASE
OF OVEREALOUS SQIRRELS'

Dr. Pecan's Wonder Elixir and the Curious Case of Overzealous Squirrels

Background: Dr. Mortimer Pecan is a man of transitions. His journey commenced in the fields as a humble pecan farmer, but life took a twist when he moved into the uncharted territories of pharmaceutical innovations, adopting the role of an unconventional pharmacist. Innovative and entrepreneurial, Dr. Pecan filed his niche in developing a potent health drink he not so modestly named 'Dr. Pecan's Wonder Elixir'. Garnering attention and raising eyebrows, he vociferously avowed that his creation has the capability to transcend the realms of natural health products, boasting a boost in memory recall, enhanced stamina, and surprisingly, improved talent for solving complex arithmetic problems. Paying homage to his roots, Dr. Pecan chose pecan extract as the powerhouse ingredient of his miraculous elixir, a testament to its natural potency.

The "Research": With an intention to carve out a niche in the ever-expanding and competitive health drink industry, Dr. Pecan took to funding his bespoke research study, aimed at substantiating the miraculous effects of his wonder elixir. The subjects deemed fit for this eclectic study were a motley crew of squirrels found in his verdant backyard, acting as willing participants (even if unknowingly so). In his perspective, who could better appreciate and showcase the nutritive benefits of a pecan-based beverage than these nut-loving creatures themselves?

Astounding Research Findings: The results of Dr. Pecan's distinctive research were nothing short of sensational. The squirrels who were administered doses of his innovative elixir were reportedly fetching and recovering their strategically hidden acorns with unprecedented 100% accuracy. Not ending there, the squirrels also showed an inexplicably high understanding of algebra, proving to be mathematically gifted creatures. This somewhat unique and unconventional study concluded with a ringing endorsement of the potent 'Dr. Pecan's Wonder Elixir', proposing its benefits for both squirrels and people across the globe.

The Unraveling of Facts: However, upon stringent scrutiny by the discerning public and a couple of perplexed scientists, a series of conspicuous discrepancies tumbled out of the closet. The towering flaws were:

1. *Bias, bias everywhere*: A taint in the purity of the research came to light when it was revealed that the pivotal study was conducted by none other than Dr. Pecan's cousin, Ms. Almond. There aren't any surprises left for guessing where her loyalties would naturally gravitate towards.

2. *Controversial Funding*: The financial support fueling this so-called groundbreaking research was a one-man show. Solely coming from the sales of Dr. Pecan's past venture, the unconventional Pecan-Infused Socks (which, undeniably, crashed and burned in the aggressive market).

3. *Restricted Diversity in Subjects*: The choice of study participants raised eyebrows and questions. As charismatic as they are, the eating habits and cognitive preferences of squirrels hardly find a parallel with the homo sapiens.

4. *Mysterious Research Methods*: Curiously, the research did not have a control group. The absence of such a crucial element, raised questions on the authenticity of the results – were the pecan-deprived squirrels just as gifted in locating their acorn stash or mastering algebra?

Concluding Observations:

Despite the commendable enthusiasm that Dr. Pecan exhibited for his innovative, nutty elixir, this scenario underscored the potential pitfalls of the domineering influence of vested interests, the paramount necessity of diverse and unbiased funding, the importance of transparency in research practices, and appropriate selection of research subjects. This example thus serves as a one-of-a-kind, nutty reminder that extraordinary research claims should be examined thoroughly before being accepted at face value.

P.S.: There remains a standing invitation to notify the academic community, should you stumble upon any squirrels solving algebra problem sets because that would be nothing short of a ground-breaking scientific discovery!

Chapter 10: Pursuing Independence - Strategies for Objective Research

Commonly known as "Big Pharma", this formidable force is often perceived as a looming titan, lurking just behind that elusive roommate who has an irritating habit of pilfering your precious peanut butter. These pharmaceutical giants cast a long and imposing shadow that can seem to outrageously overpower the illumination provided by authentic and meaningful research. The influence they wield is staggering, seemingly dwarfing attempts to explore and understand the pressing medical issues that impact all of life. Now, permit your mind to indulge me for a moment, and conjure an illustrative analogy:

You're an aspiring cook, incredibly enthusiastic about your delightful culinary creations. In order to gain some priceless feedback, you make the decision to extend an invitation to two individuals, requesting their esteemed presence for a review of your gastronomic wonders. Person One is a confidant, a precious friend of yours who, quite conveniently, and perhaps irrelevantly, still owes you a substantial sum. Person Two, on the other hand, is a pursuing professional who dedicates their life to exploring diverse culinary experiences, ever ready to provide their expert and unfiltered judgement on any dish placed in front of them; in essence, they're a food critic. In this scenario, it is fairly evident whose opinion you would be more inclined to trust, isn't it?

An absorbing scientific study carried out by Lundh et al., 2017, mirrors this situation in its findings. It revealed that analyses, which are funded by the industry, have been found to be almost six times as likely to report favorably on their own products, when compared to independent research work. This striking discrepancy exposes the heart of the problem that we're wrestling with — the tricky balancing act of lucrative financial demands and the sacred pursuit of irreproachable objective inquiry.

Back in the halcyon days of the '00s, during the captivating journey of my graduate school years, I too fell under the beguiling spell of influence — albeit the rhythmic allure of Eminem, the Backstreet Boys, and Rihanna. But that's a tantalizing tale that deserves its own dedicated time and place for telling. Importantly, the progression of meaningful research demands that we set ourselves free from the hypnotic beams cast by the singular source of commercial backing. It solicits a comprehensive shift in approach: A wholehearted embrace of diverse funding avenues instead of exclusively relying on the abyss of financial support that's offered by industry stakeholders.

The inclusion of more contributors —think government support in addition to the ample amount provided by deep-pocketed corporations— can result in a broader sample pool. It's akin to inviting not just your immediate family, but your entire community to your eagerly anticipated summer BBQ. This might be the key to obtaining external validity that would otherwise remain inaccessible via the limited reach of industry trials.

Moreover, support from foundations and academic investment introduces an element of unpredictability— it's kind of like having that eccentric aunt and uncle who are infamous for bringing along their unexpected yet always impressively delightful dishes. So, we could definitely use more of that bolstering of impartiality in scientific pursuits!

Remember that one time when I had toiled to elucidate upon the intriguing topic of "The Impact of Socks with Sandals on Cognitive Function"? My hard work was unfortunately received with much less than the expected applause, as some dispiriting results were mysteriously excised from the final report.

Where mandatory outcome registration and transparent analysis would have come to the rescue, without censorship, my fashion-forward subjects would have been saved from obscurity. They would have countered and closed the gap presented by publication bias, which often seeks to hide undesirable outcomes (Turner et al., 2008).

Pre-registration can be perceived as making a declaration to your friends about baking a sweet, luscious cake for them, and then, without any sort of subterfuge or sleight of hand, not sneaking in a pie instead. By instilling this integrity of methodology before the commencement of data collection, we uphold the honesty of the research process.

Furthermore, embracing collaborative designs is a pivotal practice for research. It's like organizing a potluck - inviting everyone to the table to share their unique perspectives and delicious contributions. The more diverse the participants, the richer and more balanced the findings we can derive.

Finally, at the heart of this entire endeavor are the patients. They're the precious beneficiaries of the relentless tug of war between research needs and financial interests. These beloved individuals deserve to be serenaded with an empowering symphony of helpful information, which would guide them towards making autonomous decisions about their healthcare journey. Conclusively, to continue the analogy, prioritizing independence above influence could be likened to choosing a slice of your grandma's homemade pie (bursting with love) over a commercially packaged dessert. This approach will invariably lead to a better serving for those who rely on research to determine their healthcare choices for maximizing their overall wellbeing.

Conclusively, with a collective will, coherent collaboration, and perhaps-a-catchy-tune-or-two, objective evidence can light up the path for everyone who ventures upon it freely. And, as I often say, the journey is always more enjoyable when you have a comfortable pair of shoes (preferably, not accompanied by socks with sandals).

Time for Reflection:

1. **Industry Influence vs. Independence:** Reflect on a time when you've seen or experienced biases in decision-making, whether in a personal, academic, or professional setting. How might these biases compare to the potential influence of industry funding on research outcomes?

2. **Diverse Funding Sources:** Why might a research study funded by multiple, diverse sources (like governments, foundations, and academic institutions) be viewed as more credible or unbiased than one funded by a single commercial entity? Can you think of any real-world scenarios or products where diverse funding might have altered public opinion?

3. **Transparency and Integrity:** Consider the importance of pre-registration and collaborative designs in research. Why do you think transparency in methods and collaboration in design might lead to more trustworthy results? Have you ever encountered a situation where knowing the process behind a decision made it more trustworthy?

4. **Patient Empowerment:** How do you feel when making decisions based on well-researched information versus decisions made in the absence of such information? Drawing from the chapter, why might it be crucial for patients to have access to independent and transparent research when determining their care options?

References

Elbe, S., & Caraça, J. (2020). Rethinking global health governance in an era of multiple crises. Global Policy, 11(1), 1-9.

Lundh, A., Lexchin, J., Mintzes, B., Schroll, J. B., & Bero, L. (2017). Industry sponsorship and research outcome. Cochrane Database of Systematic Reviews, 2.

Schor, E. L. (2011). Policymaking in schools of medicine as viewed through the lens of pharmaceutical marketing. Academic Medicine, 86(2), 129-134.

Storebø, O. J., Ramstad, E., Krogh, H. B., Nilausen, T. D., Skoog, M., Holmskov, M., ... & Moreira-Maia, C. R. (2018).

Methylphenidate for children and adolescents with attention deficit hyperactivity disorder (ADHD). Cochrane Database of Systematic Reviews, (2).

Turner, E. H., Matthews, A. M., Linardatos, E., Tell, R. A., & Rosenthal, R. (2008). Selective publication of antidepressant trials and its influence on apparent efficacy. New England Journal of Medicine, 358(3), 252-260.

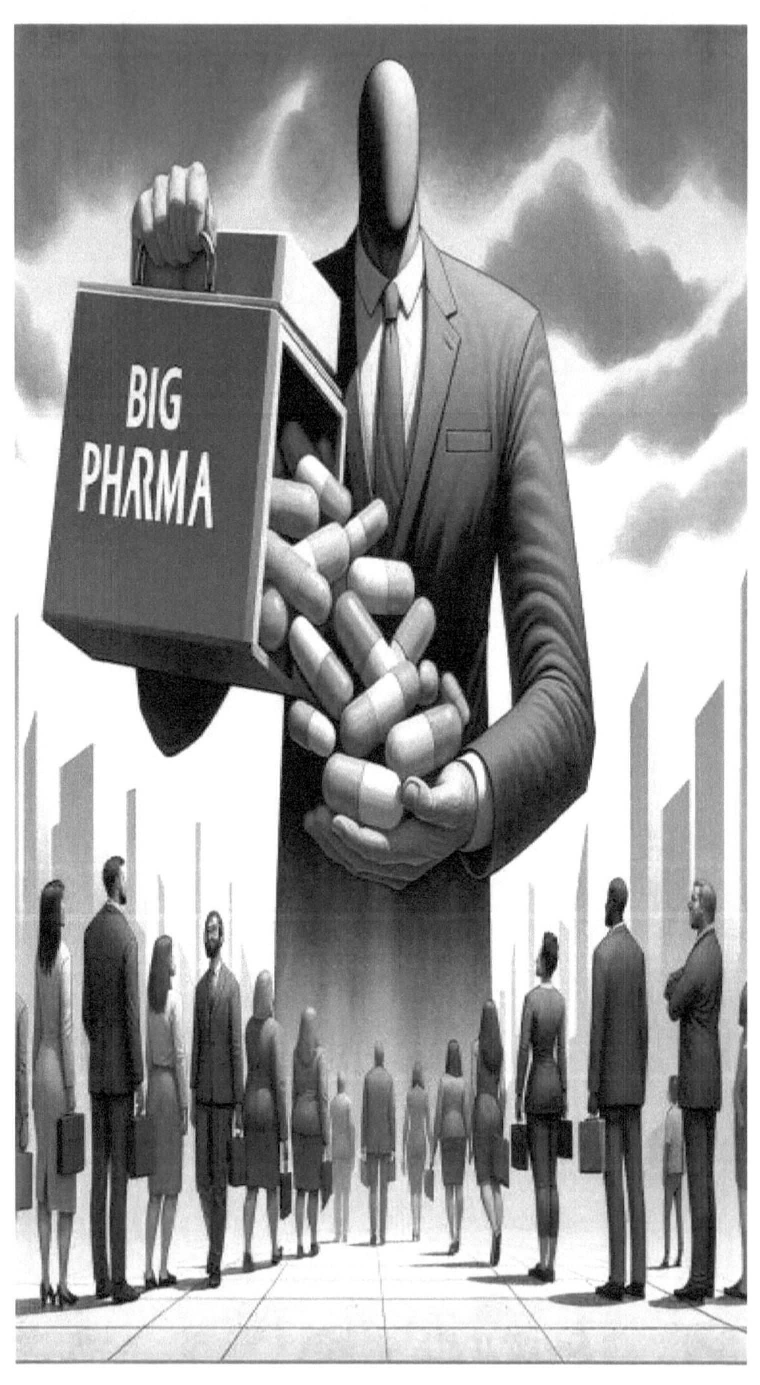

BIG
PHARMA

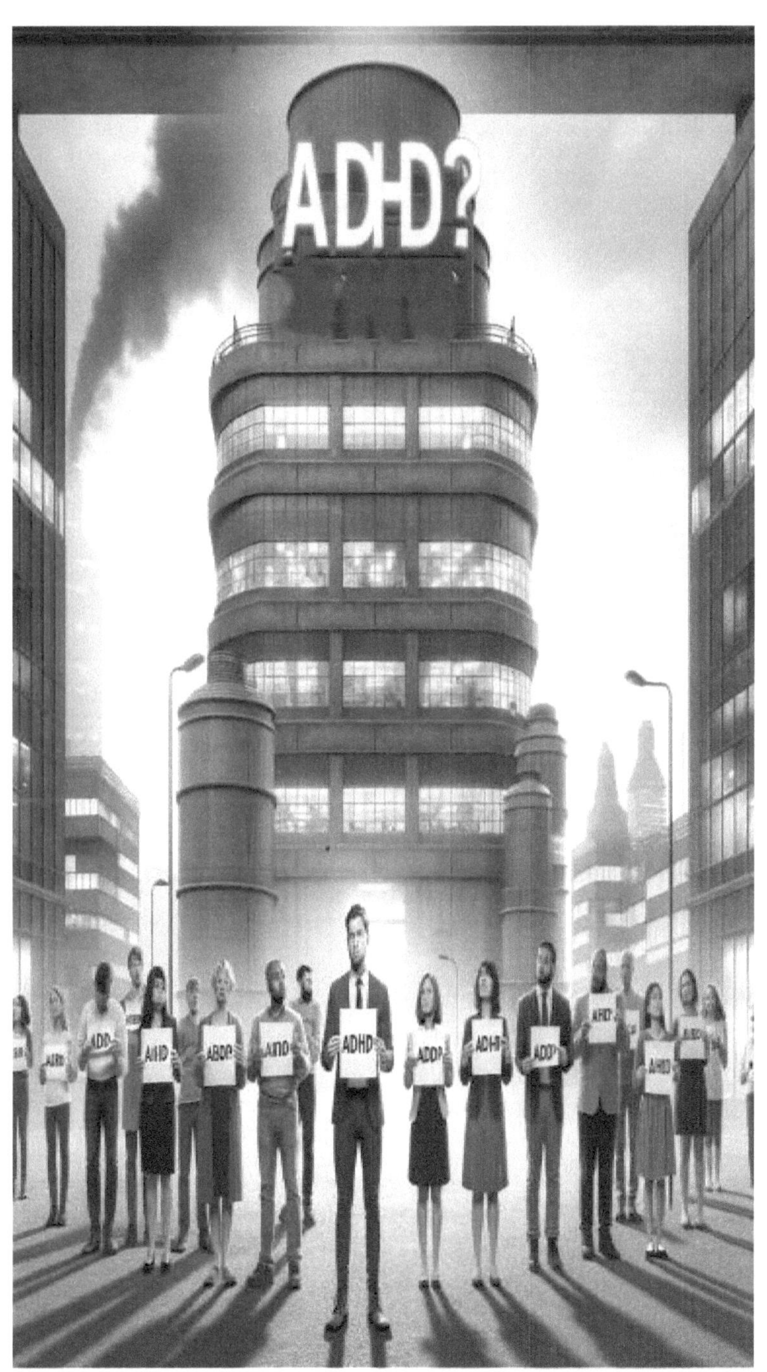

ADHD?

Beyond "Big Pharma Says You Have ADHD!"

As we reach the conclusion of "Big Pharma Says You Have ADHD!", it is clear the journey through the chapters has been both eye-opening and challenging. Through a series of carefully crafted anecdotal stories and in-depth explorations, this book has provided a critical lens on the complex and often controversial interactions between the pharmaceutical industry and the ADHD narrative.

In "The Tale of Daydreaming Danny and the Mysterious Marketing Magicians", we began by uncovering how the ADHD narrative is shaped by powerful pharmaceutical companies. This theme, echoed throughout this book, set the stage for a deeper understanding of the intricate dance between marketing, medicine, and mental health.

As we progressed to "The Curious Case of Greg and the 'Distract-a-lot' Syndrome", we witnessed how awareness campaigns, often funded by Big Pharma, can influence public perception and understanding of ADHD. This influence, as revealed in the subsequent chapters, extends deeply into the medicalization of ADHD, diagnostic criteria, and the very definition of the condition.

The stories of Dr. Green, Dr. Larry, and Tim illuminated the subtle yet significant ways in which pharmaceutical companies shape the diagnosis and treatment of ADHD. These narratives brought to life the risks associated with direct-to-consumer (DTC) advertising and the potential for misdiagnosis or overdiagnosis driven by commercial interests.

"The Great Guacamole Gala of 2023" and the tale of Dr. Monty highlighted the often-overlooked influence of industry partnerships and the impact of pharmaceutical marketing on healthcare providers. These chapters underscored the importance of maintaining a critical eye on the information we receive and the sources from which it comes.

The global reach of Big Pharma, as illustrated in "The Curious Case of Bubbly Billy in Bhutan", reminds us that this is not just a localized issue but a worldwide concern. The story of Dr. Phil McCrackin's involvement with "PillPal" promos and Dr. Pecan's adventures brought us face-to-face with the need for stringent regulation and objective research in the field of ADHD and mental health.

Throughout this book, we have explored the multifaceted relationship between Big Pharma and the ADHD narrative. It is a relationship fraught with ethical dilemmas, conflicts of interest, and significant implications for public health and individual well-being.

However, this book is not just a critique; it is a call to action. It urges us to be vigilant and informed consumers of medical information. It encourages healthcare professionals to critically examine the sources of their knowledge and the potential biases that may influence their practice. It calls for stricter regulations to curb the undue influence of pharmaceutical companies on healthcare. And importantly, it advocates for independent and objective research to guide our understanding of ADHD and its treatment.

In closing, "Big Pharma Says You Have ADHD!" is not just a commentary on the state of ADHD diagnosis and treatment; it is a rallying cry for a more informed, ethical, and patient-centered approach to mental health. As readers, you are now equipped with the knowledge and perspective to question, challenge, and contribute to the ongoing discourse around ADHD and the broader implications of pharmaceutical influence in healthcare. Together, we can strive towards a future where health decisions are made based on unbiased information and the genuine well-being of individuals, free from the overshadowing influence of commercial interests.

Thank you for embarking on this enlightening journey. May it inspire continued learning, critical thinking, and positive change.

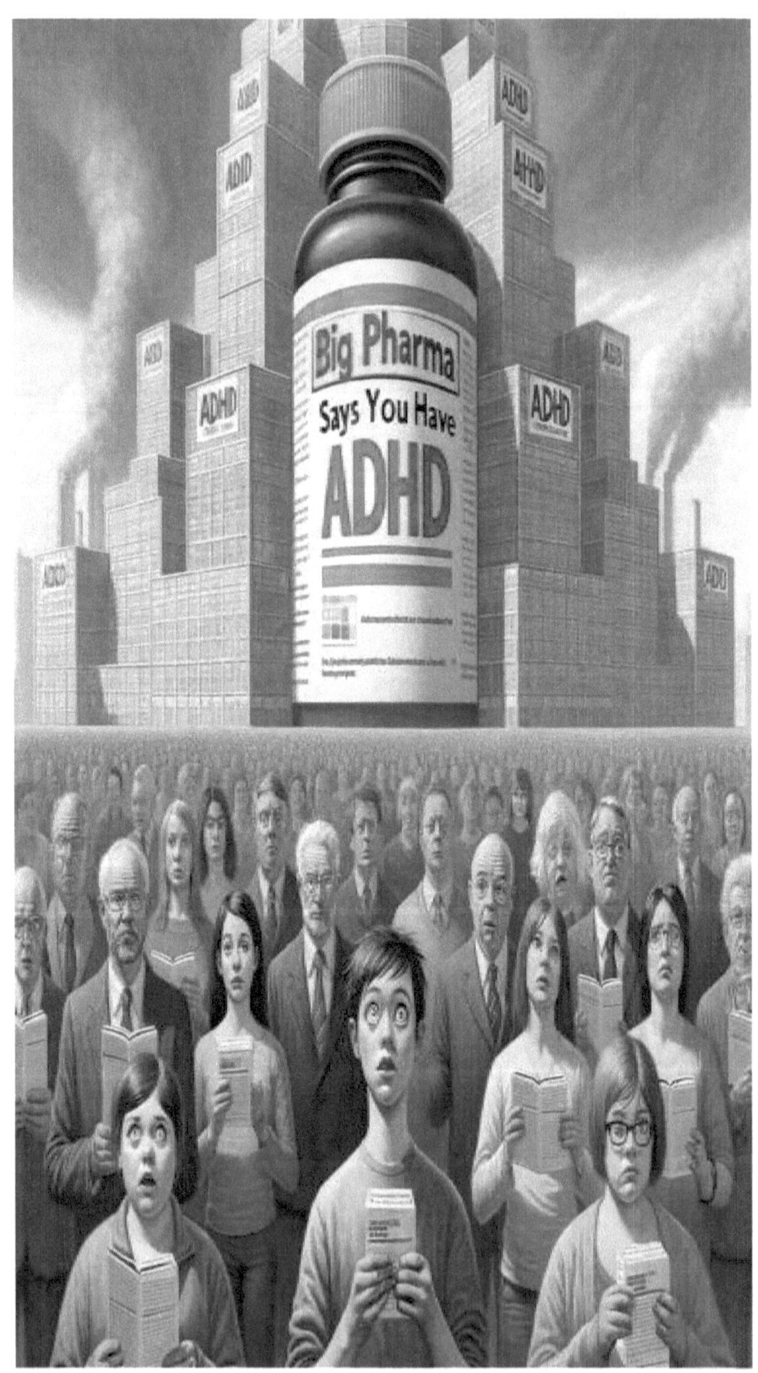
Big Pharma
Says You Have
ADHD
ADHD
ADHD
ADHD
ADHD
ADHD
ADHD

www.ingramcontent.com/pod-product-compliance
Lightning Source LLC
Chambersburg PA
CBHW051308250726
48656CB00004B/1544